Birthing Positions

~ Dedicated to my wonderful children
Victoria and Daniel ~

Birthing Positions

What do women want?
Do midwives know best?

Regina Coppen

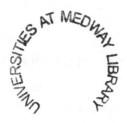

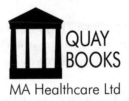

QUAY
BOOKS

MA Healthcare Ltd

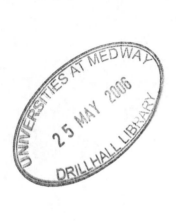

Quay Books Division, MA Healthcare Limited, St Jude's Church, Dulwich Road,
London SE24 0PB

British Library Cataloguing-in-Publication Data
A catalogue record is available for this book

© MA Healthcare Limited 2005
ISBN 1 85642 256 9

Printed in Great Britain by Ashford Colour Press Ltd, Gosport, Hants

Contents

'One must learn by doing the thing, for though you think you know it, you have no certainty until you try.'

Sophocles, 400 BC

(Could the great philosopher, Sophocles be referring to the use of the upright position, and the importance of encouraging midwives and women to try it before rejecting the idea?)

Acknowledgements

I would like to thank all the women and midwives who participated in my study for their faithful encouragement, without which this book would not have been possible. I salute you.

To all future mothers-to-be, I hope this book will stir and move mountains for you regarding your choice of birthing positions in labour. I wish you well.

To all my students, I hope you will learn much, practise hard and listen fervently to what women want – to do this, you must first ask them.

To my dear friends Dr Gill Aston, Jane Bott, Anne Brown, Margaret and Douglas Excell and my niece Elizabeth – thank you for putting so much faith in me to complete this book!

Finally, to my dearest sister Patricia, who is always so proud of my achievements even before I have completed them, thank you for your unfailing love and support.

Foreword

It may come as a surprise to readers that something as fundamental to human life as birthing positions should be surrounded by controversy. Yet, as this book so clearly indicates, it is. Dr Regina Coppen, herself an experienced midwife, takes the reader through the issues and then reports on a study that attempts to address the matter for the twenty-first century. As a result, everyone involved in the outcome and potential hazards of natural body processes would benefit from reading this book – whether they have experienced, or are about to experience, the event; or whether they are responsible for providing care and support to those who will.

The first point that emerges from a careful reading of historical sources is that different cultures may provide lessons that challenge assumptions underpinning current obstetric or midwifery practices. Although giving birth is necessary for the survival of the species, what Dr Coppen illustrates is that one should not ignore the varied ways in which women over the centuries have responded instinctively to the delivery of their baby.

The second point that emerges from the literature is that antenatal education may not, if general in content, give women the authority to make their own choices, even if they are given the opportunity. It is too easy to forget that professionals – in this case, midwives – not only represent a 'power figure' who can inhibit joint decision-making, but they also need themselves to be committed to alternative practices.

Is there a way forward? Dr Coppen thinks there is – but only if, during antenatal education, the information provided focuses directly on the issues about which women are invited to make choices, and if they are helped to engage in joint decision-making. In Part 2, Dr Coppen reports the results of a study that tested this hypothesis. The research is important not only because of the findings, but also because of the technique used: a randomised controlled trial (RCT), long considered the 'gold standard' for evaluating the effectiveness of procedures. All midwives would be wise to reflect on the findings, since they show how difficult it can be to ensure that women's choices are respected throughout the birth process. Clearly, further research will be needed to uncover the underlying reasons why women's decision-making during the second stage of delivery broke down, but the midwives' own knowledge-base may also need to be challenged.

The message, then, seems to be that a more focused antenatal-education programme can help a woman to be more involved during the birth of her baby, albeit with limitations. Even so, education classes alone will not secure success. Midwives themselves need to be committed to evidence-based practice so that, despite their own preferences, they recognise the effectiveness of other delivery methods. Hopefully, this excellent book will go some way to achieving what the Department of Health, in 2005, set as a standard to be achieved:

... a woman should be able to choose the most appropriate place and professional to attend during childbirth, based on her wishes and cultural preferences and any medical and obstetric needs that she or her baby may have.

Professor Rosemary Crow,
Emeritus of Surrey University, England,
and Honorary Professor of Nursing,
Dublin City University, Ireland,
August 2005

Section 1

CHAPTER 1

Definitions of recumbent and upright positions for childbirth

There is no universally agreed definition of recumbent and upright positions for childbirth. Many health professionals cannot agree on a definition; furthermore, as soon became clear to the author while reviewing the literature, definitions of these terms also vary between authors, doctors, midwives, laypersons and researchers, and from one study to the next. The term 'alternative position' has also been used by midwives and women to describe a form of upright position such as the 'all-fours' position. This book will therefore begin by defining recumbent and upright positions for childbirth, to provide clarity, consistency and a better understanding of the terms.

The terms 'recumbent position' and 'alternative position' can be ambiguous and mean different things to different practitioners. For example, in a qualitative study, Coppen (1997) evaluated midwives' knowledge of birth positions by asking 10 midwives from three clinical settings in London to describe what they understood by the term 'recumbent position'. The midwives described several positions, ranging from delivering in a horizontal position, sometimes termed 'flat in bed', to delivering on one's side (lateral), to delivering in the lithotomy position (lying down with the legs supported by stirrups). Some midwives were not aware that the conventional birth position – a sitting posture supported by a wedge or several pillows on the bed – is described in the literature as a form of recumbent position, either semi-recumbent, dorsal-recumbent or supported supine position (Humphrey et al, 1973; Dundes, 1987; Johnstone et al, 1987; Dunn, 1991; Waldenstrom and Gottval, 1991; Kelly et al, 1999). Furthermore, in the systematic reviews by Nikodem (1995) and Gupta and Nikodem (2000a), the semi-recumbent position was categorised as an upright position and compared with other recumbent positions!

It is argued that the semi-recumbent position cannot possibly be termed an upright position because of its low-lying posture. Many midwives point out that the semi-recumbent position does little to enhance women's progress in labour. It is also a position that often causes women to slip down the bed when pushing during the second stage of labour, resulting in them delivering 'flat on their back', against the force of gravity.

Further confusion is caused by the use of the term 'sitting position' by some researchers and midwifery practitioners to describe a woman delivering in an upright position on a birthing chair (Cottrell and Shannahan, 1986, 1987; Liu, 1986; Gardosi et al, 1989a; Crowley et al, 1991), whereas others refer to the sitting position as a semi-recumbent position (Gupta and Nikodem 2000a, Rosser 2003), thereby compounding the meaning of the term. The semi-recumbent position is often called the conventional position. Moreover, some midwives define alternative position as any position other than the recumbent or conventional positions.

What, then, is the conventional birthing position today, and is the use of a birthing chair or stool considered an alternative position? Bodner-Adler et al (2003) defined the upright position as free squatting or any alternative position. For clarity, therefore, it is argued that 'recumbent position' and 'semi-recumbent position' should not be confused with the 'upright sitting posture' or 'sitting position' described by some midwives (Coppen, 1997). Indeed, there appears to be no agreement among professionals and researchers on what distinguishes upright from non-upright positions, or alternative from recumbent positions (Humphrey et al, 1973; Dundes, 1987; Johnstone et al, 1987; Dunn, 1991; Kelly et al, 1999; Nikodem, 1995; Gupta and Nikodem, 2000a; Bodner-Adler et al, 2003).

The parameters for the various positions need to be clearly defined to avoid further confusion and 'muddying' of the different terminologies. I suggest that the term 'alternative position' is vague and should be avoided as much as possible, as it only adds to the plethora of untenable definitions that already exist in the literature.

For the purpose of this book, therefore, the term **upright position** will refer to any of the following:

º   Sitting upright with weight on the buttocks, back elevated *greater than* 45° from the horizontal, on or off the bed, with or without the aid of birth cushions and mattress. The emphasis here is that the woman must be kept upright at an angle greater than 45°. The partner or birth attendant can play an important role in supporting the woman in this position (*Figure 1.1*)

º   Sitting on a birthing chair (*Figures 1.2a–c*)

º   Sitting on a birth stool or stone (*Figure 1.3*)

º   Kneeling-crouching position (*Figures 1.4a & b*)

○   Squatting position *(Figure 1.5)*
○   Semi-squatting position – this lies between the standing position and the full squat, where the woman may rest both hands on her thighs with knees bent for support or, when leaning over the bed or chair, with knees bent; also known as suspended squat, normally with hands around her partner's neck *(Figures 1.6a & b)*
○   Hanging on to a rope in a squatting or semi-squatting position *(Figure 1.7)*
○   Kneeling position *(Figure 1.8a–c)*
○   'All-fours' position (also known as the 'hands and knees' position) *(Figure 1.9)*
○   Standing position *(Figure 1.10)*.

The ***recumbent position*** will refer to any of the following:

○   Semi-recumbent position – achieved by the use of pillows or wedge on a delivery bed with the back resting at an angle of less than or equal to 30°, with or without a footrest. This is the conventional position commonly used today *(Figure 1.11)*.
○   Lithotomy position – lying on the back with both legs suspended and supported by an attendant or, more commonly today, stirrups *(Figure 1.12)*.
○   Recumbent, dorsal or supine position – lying down on the bed, with face upwards, with or without head support *(Figure 1.13)*.
○   Lateral or Sim's lateral position – delivering on the left side, lying down with right leg raised *(Figure 1.14)*.

Examples of upright birthing positions (*Figures 1.1–1.10*)

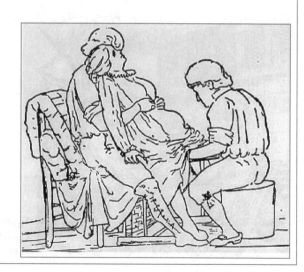

Figure 1.1:
Sitting upright with partner
support, showing how modesty
and privacy are preserved.

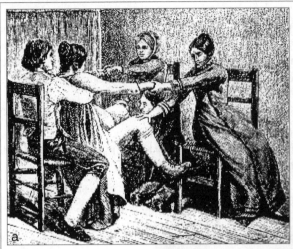

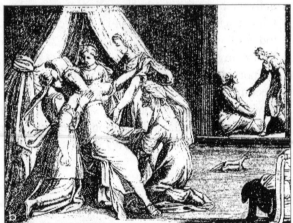

Figures 1.2a & b:
Upright posture on a chair
with several attendants.

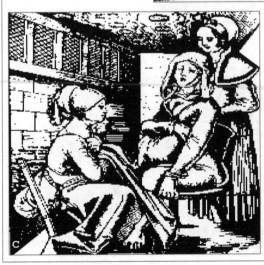

Figure 1.2c:
Upright posture on a chair,
leaning on an accoucheur.

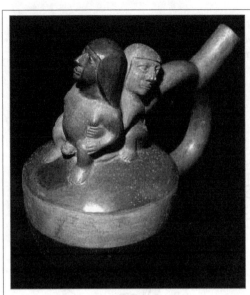

Figure 1.3:
Obstetric scene depicted on a terracotta water jug, Peru. The midwife is shown sitting behind the mother, assisting with the delivery of the child.

Figure 1.4a (below):
A woman in the kneeling-crouching position.

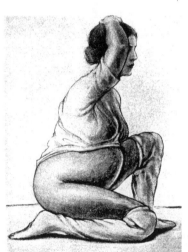

Figure 1.4b (above):
A woman in the kneeling-crouching position.

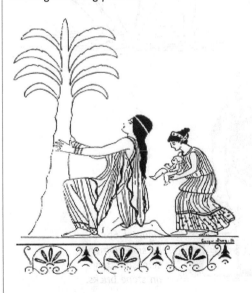

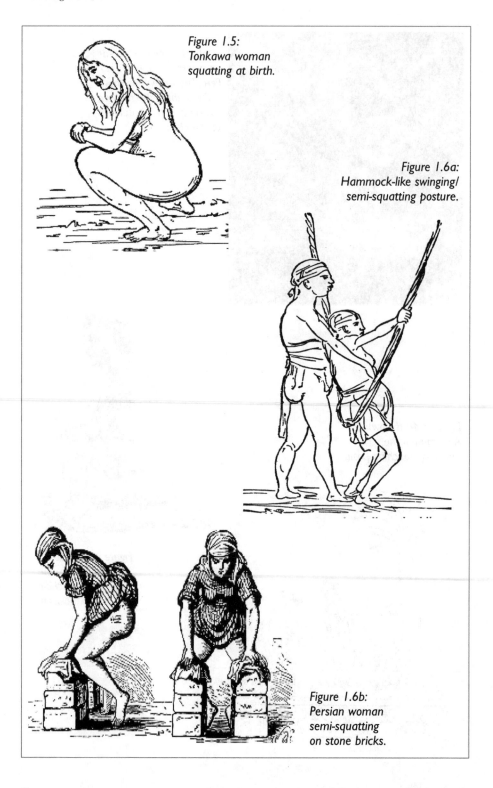

Figure 1.5:
Tonkawa woman
squatting at birth.

Figure 1.6a:
Hammock-like swinging/
semi-squatting posture.

Figure 1.6b:
Persian woman
semi-squatting
on stone bricks.

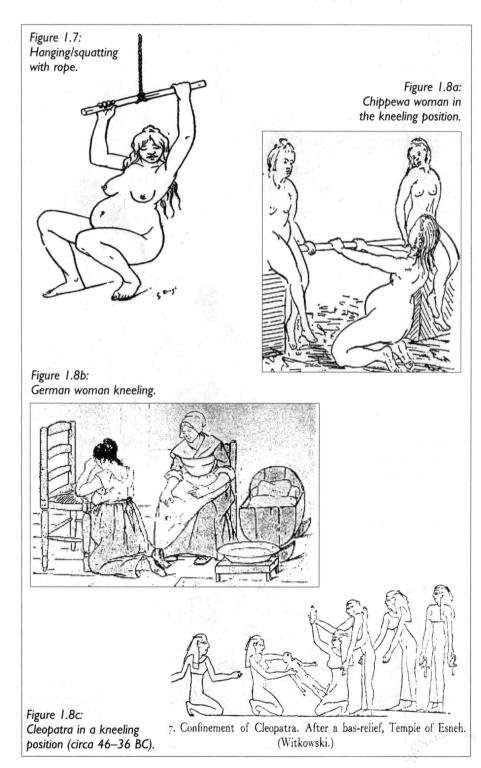

Figure 1.7:
Hanging/squatting
with rope.

Figure 1.8a:
Chippewa woman in
the kneeling position.

Figure 1.8b:
German woman kneeling.

Figure 1.8c:
Cleopatra in a kneeling
position (circa 46–36 BC).

7. Confinement of Cleopatra. After a bas-relief, Temple of Esneh.
(Witkowski.)

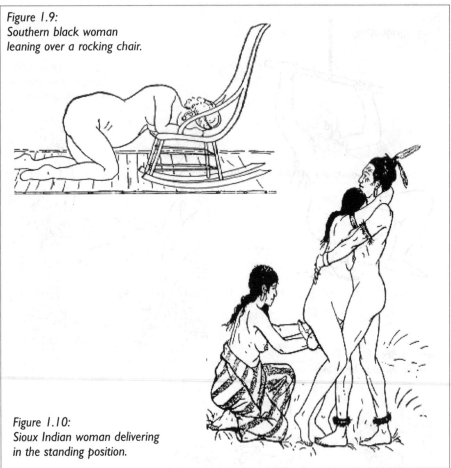

Figure 1.9:
Southern black woman
leaning over a rocking chair.

Figure 1.10:
Sioux Indian woman delivering
in the standing position.

Examples of recumbent birthing positions (*Figures 1.11–1.14*)

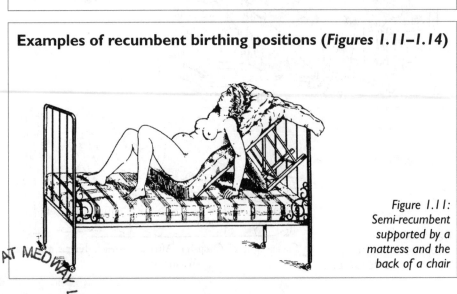

Figure 1.11:
Semi-recumbent
supported by a
mattress and the
back of a chair

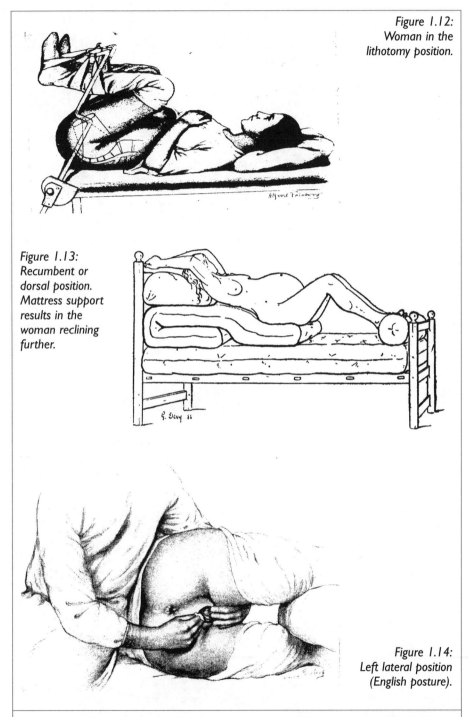

Figure 1.12:
Woman in the lithotomy position.

Figure 1.13:
Recumbent or dorsal position. Mattress support results in the woman reclining further.

Figure 1.14:
Left lateral position (English posture).

Figures 1.1–1.14 are reproduced by kind permission of Dr John Jarcho MD (30 March 2002). Legends adapted by Dr Regina Coppen.

CHAPTER 2

Background and introduction

Choice of birthing position receives scant attention in both the public and the clinical arenas today. Unlike hotly debated issues, such as the escalating rate of caesarean section, whether to choose a hospital or home birth, and the use of controversial technologies to increase fecundity or fertility, asking women and professionals their views on birthing positions does not have the same urgency. Yet, when it comes to choice and decision-making, such a low profile clinical issue can suddenly become contentious and controversial.

Little is known about the synergy that exists between the woman's and the midwife's choice of birthing positions and the factors involved when mothers do not deliver in their position of choice. Some midwives may believe that as long as the outcome is a healthy normal baby, it does not matter whether a woman delivers on the bed, off the bed, or in a recumbent or an upright position. However, I beg to differ in defence of women's right to choose, be informed and deliver in the birthing position of their choice. This book will demonstrate the importance of identifying with women in their personal birth choices, and will highlight a tried and tested method, namely the provision of *focused information* on the benefits of upright birthing positions to aid women's decision-making, which midwives can apply to encourage women to deliver in the upright position.

I will begin by reviewing past and present cultural norms regarding birthing positions. The aim is to enhance understanding of the different childbirth positions used in practice today. A discourse on the scientific evidence for the use of upright positions will be presented, and the current state of antenatal education will be discussed to illustrate the need to include practical sessions on birthing positions for women in preparation for childbirth.

Past and present cultural norms – timeline

Women have been delivering in upright positions for centuries. The earliest record of birthing in an upright position dates back to 5000 BC, in biblical notations (Exodus 1:16), when midwives helped women to deliver on birth stools, through to an Egyptian drawing clearly depicting birth in a squatting position (Jarcho, 1934; Russell, 1982). Contemporary descriptions of women delivering in upright positions are less overt; for example, when birth is portrayed in the media, especially in popular dramas, the recumbent position appears to be the norm. However, the evidence will show that women prefer to use the upright birthing position and, given the choice, will adopt what they consider to be the most natural position for them. The evidence will also show that women consider birthing in the upright position to be the natural position (Rigby, 1857; Jarcho, 1934; De Jong et al, 1997; Coppen, 2002).

A timeline charting the historical progression of recumbent *vs* upright birthing positions can be constructed from published works (*Table 2.1*). In some cases, the country of origin, or different cultural groups using the positions, are highlighted. In the absence of published papers, evidence from illustrations has been included in the timeline.

TABLE 2.1: Timeline charting the historical progression of recumbent *vs* upright birthing positions

Publication or author	Place or cultural group	Timeline	Recumbent position	Upright position
The Bible	Egypt, Mediterranean	5000 BC		Squatting and semi-squatting, birth stools
Weindler (1915) Mayer (1942) Alaily (1996) Housholder (1974)	Egypt – evidence seen in medical papyri	1450 BC		Birth stools, chair, kneeling
Hippocrates De Lee (1934) Thompson (1957)	Greece	Circa 420 BC		Recommended the obstetric chair
Cleopatra's birth illustrated	Egypt	46–36 BC		Kneeling position
Shorter (1991)	Western society	AD 1000–1530		Standing, squatting
Inca tribes (*Figure 1.3*)	South America	AD 1100–1530		Kneeling, squatting
Fasbender (1906)	Ephesus	2nd century AD		Birth stools
Naroll et al (1961)	Primitive cultures	Circa 13th–12th century		Squatting, kneeling, suspended on poles – standing or swinging on a hammock

Shorter (1991)	German cities	14th–15th century		Birth stools
Shorter (1991)	Central Europe	16th century		Birth stools (city women), standing or squatting (rural women)
Alaily (1996)	Cairo	16th–17th century		Marble stone delivery stools
Alaily (1996)	Holland, France, US	Early 18th century		Wooden birthing chairs
Shorter (1991)	England – middle and upper classes	Mid-18th century	Left lateral or dorsal position (preferred by doctors)	Kneeling position (preferred by midwives)
Rigby (1857)	England	19th century		Kneeling, squatting, standing (when left alone without medical intervention)
Englemann (1882)	Western society	19th century	Supine, prone, dorsal	
Shorter (1991)	England	19th century	Left lateral	
Shorter (1991)	Bavaria, Switzerland	Early 19th century		Squatting or supported with slings or vertical ropes
Alaily (1996)	Egyptians, Japan	19th century		Birth chairs
Coffin (1995)	England	19th century	Left lateral	
Jarcho (1929)	Asiatic, mid-Eastern, Eastern, South American population	16th–19th century		Standing, kneeling, squatting, semi-squatting, crouching
Jarcho (1929)	Western population	20th century	Recumbent, semi-recumbent	Chair – sitting position
Hewes (1957)	Western population	Early 20th century	Recumbent, semi-recumbent	
Hewes (1957)	Asiatic and Eastern population	Early 20th century		Standing and squatting or crouching
Atwood (1976)	Non-Western cultures	19th century		Standing, sitting squatting, kneeling
Shorter (1991)	American society	Early to mid-20th century	Lithotomy	
Waldenstrom and Gottval (1991)	England	Late 20th century	Recumbent, semi-recumbent	To a lesser extent, birth stools
Alaily (1996)	Switzerland, Holland	Late 20th century		Parturition chairs, stools
Coppen (2002)	England	Present day	Semi-recumbent	To a lesser extent, kneeling, all fours, standing

There is clear evidence from the timeline that the use of upright positions was commonplace from biblical times until about the 18th century, when the incumbent medical practitioners (mostly male doctors) began to intervene with the natural childbirth process in the guise that women needed help with delivering their babies. No doubt a small percentage of women do require medical assistance, but 'the law of nature' suggests that the majority of women are quite capable of delivering their babies naturally without medical intervention, as shown clearly in this timeline. Interestingly, women from the Asiatic and Mediterranean countries, and certain European countries such as Holland and Switzerland, have continued to adopt the upright position for delivery to the present day. The historical perspective of birthing positions will be discussed in more detail in Chapter 3.

Scientific evidence on the use of upright birthing positions

A systematic review of all available scientific journals found only 25 randomised controlled trials (RCTs) that compared the use of the upright and recumbent positions (Chan, 1963; Humphrey et al, 1973; McManus and Calder, 1978; Calder et al, 1983; Martilla et al, 1983; Stewart et al, 1983; Liddell and Fisher, 1985; Hemminki et al, 1986; Turner et al, 1986; Chen et al, 1987; Johnstone et al, 1987; Liu, 1988; Gardosi et al, 1989a, 1989b; Gupta et al, 1989a; Stewart and Spiby, 1989a; Crowley et al, 1991; Radkey et al, 1991; Waldenstrom and Gottval, 1991; Allahbadia and Vaidya, 1991; Bhardwaj, 1994; Kafka et al, 1994; De Jong et al, 1997; Bomfim-Hyppolito, 1998; Racinet et al, 1999). Before this systematic review, only two reviews comparing the upright and recumbent positions had been published in the Cochrane Database of systematic reviews. The second publication (Gupta and Nikodem, 2000a) was updated to include two further RCTs from the original review of 16 RCTs (Nikodem, 1995).

Such paucity of interest may be due to the assumed benefits of the recumbent or semi-recumbent position, or the innate assumption that women will be able to articulate and ask for whatever position they prefer. These systematic reviews clearly demonstrate that the upright position is superior to the recumbent position during the second stage of labour. In particular, the evidence showed that when the upright birthing position was used, fewer women experienced severe pain at birth, the incidence of abnormal fetal heart rate patterns was reduced, the second stage of labour was shorter, fewer women needed assisted deliveries, and fewer episiotomies were performed. These advantages outweighed the only two disadvantages found, namely that some women sustained blood loss greater than 500 ml and some women experienced increased second-degree perineal tears (Gupta and Hofmeyr, 2004).

Yet in clinical practice today, the use of recumbent positions, particularly the semi-recumbent position, appears to be the norm. It is argued that this may be the result of women not being informed of other available options, or that obstetricians and midwives may lack the information, skills, confidence and knowledge regarding the use of upright birthing positions. Moreover, it has been assumed, without clear evidence, that most women prefer to use recumbent positions.

However, none of the RCTs reviewed sought women's specific views on the use of the various positions. Those that did address women's views included only a cursory report of these, such as their degree of satisfaction with the birth outcome (Hemminki et al, 1986; Stewart and Spiby, 1989a; Waldenstrom and Gottval, 1991). Since a positive birth outcome is often linked with a high satisfaction rate, it cannot be assumed that women's needs were necessarily met regarding their preferred choice of birthing positions. These trials neither included nor addressed specifically the issues of whether women were included in decision-making *per se*, how informed the women were, or how the decision on their choice of birthing position was made. It was argued that doubts existed as to some women's capacity to deal with the vast amount of information available to them when making decisions within the clinical arena. It is sometimes assumed that women want midwives to help them unscramble some of the decisions that have to be made. On the other hand, it could be argued that if women are not empowered with the knowledge, they cannot be expected to make an informed decision about their choice of position in labour.

It is hypothesised that one reason for the continuing trend in the use of recumbent or semi-recumbent positions is that pregnant women are not informed about the benefits of the upright position for childbirth. It is reasonable to assume that if women are unaware of the choices available to them, they cannot be expected to know what to choose, what is best for them, or how to make an informed choice of birthing positions.

It is my wish that this book will help women to make an informed decision on their choice of birthing position before they go into labour, and give women the confidence to convey their wishes to their midwives or birth professionals. I also hope that it will assist midwives and any professionals involved in caring for pregnant women, especially those in labour, in understanding what women really want regarding their choice of birthing positions. I will have succeeded in my quest to help women make an informed decision on choice of birthing position if this book has the desired effect in influencing midwives and healthcare professionals who have never delivered women in the upright posture to do so – with confidence, gusto and assurance that they are doing it because it is the right thing to do and it is what women want.

Educating women on the use of different birthing positions

Much of antenatal education today focuses on general coping mechanisms for labour, ranging from the use of medication to relaxation techniques, exercises and, to a lesser extent, posture (Hillier and Slade, 1989; Byrne-Lynch, 1991; National Childbirth Trust, 1991; Combes and Schonveld, 1992; Slade et al, 1993; Niven and Gisjbers, 1996; Oliver et al, 1996; Slade, 1996; Sagady, 2000). It is unclear whether women are able to apply what they have learnt from antenatal education when they are in labour.

Niven and Gisjbers (1996) suggested that an association between attendance at antenatal class and the use of coping strategies for labour existed only for relaxation methods. Byrne-Lynch (1991) reported that 95% of women used some form of coping strategy in early labour. Walking and upright positions were the most common strategies used in early labour in 65% of women in the study. Only 33% of women used breathing exercises to cope with labour. However, only 20% of this sample had attended classes and the study was not randomised.

Copstick et al (1985) investigated whether antenatal training was useful in helping women to cope during labour. They suggested that women do not necessarily apply what they have learnt.

Much has been written about the benefits of antenatal preparation on pain-related outcomes. Timm (1979) carried out an evaluative study, which tried to control for the effects of attendance. Women were randomly assigned to one of three conditions: standard prenatal classes, knitting classes, or no classes but encouragement to consult doctors or nurses about childbearing. Women who attended the prenatal classes used significantly less medication compared with the two control groups. However, Timm did not clarify what was taught at the prenatal classes and how it was taught, and was vague about the quality of the consultation between the women and the doctors or nurses. Moreover, it was unclear how the use of medication was recorded.

Hetherington (1990) compared 52 couples who attended childbirth classes with a control group of 203 matched for age, race, parity and marital status. Prepared couples were found to have had more spontaneous deliveries, and less analgesia or anaesthesia. Many women in this study attributed their satisfying experiences to the classes and felt that using methods taught to them in the classes had helped them to cope better. However, as this was a small study, the results cannot be generalised to the whole population.

Sagady (2000) emphasised the importance of reviewing the way that antenatal preparation is given to women, and pointed out that adequate preparation may help to reduce the high rate of caesarean section experienced by women in the USA. There is evidence to show that the provision of adequate and appropriate health information to women can reduce anxiety and is associated with higher satisfaction levels (Garrud et al, 2001; Horey et al, 2004).

McKay (1984) and Coppen (2002) argued against confining women in bed and for greater mobility in labour, encouraging women to keep upright as much as possible since the evidence shows that this would shorten their labour, reduce labour pains and give them a better chance of delivering normally. Sadly, this is not the norm in current practice, and it takes an assertive woman to keep mobile and maintain the upright posture during labour, or a midwife in favour of natural childbirth or intervention-free practice to encourage women to do this.

Lauzon and Hodnett (1998) identified one study in a Cochrane review that assessed the effects of teaching specific criteria for the self-diagnosis of active labour onset. They found that specific antenatal education programmes were associated with a reduction in the mean number of visits to the labour suite before the onset of labour. Indeed, it is not uncommon for midwives to advise women to wait as long as possible at home and labour in the comfort of their own home as long as they feel happy to do so, rather than admit themselves too early into the labour suite.

Few women are aware that the moment they step into the labour suite the 'timing' of their labour will be recorded, increasing their risk of medical intervention exponentially if their labour does not progress at a rate that is 'comfortable' for the healthcare professionals. For example, if a primigravida (a woman who is pregnant for the first time) is in labour for more than 24 hours in the labour suite, most obstetricians would be tempted to hasten labour by prescribing oxytocin (Syntocinon) to be given intravenously. Yet the decision to intervene in this way is arbitrary as there is no evidence to show that a woman having her first baby should deliver within a certain time.

I believe that many births are induced unnecessarily. Before the women know it, a cascade of intervention ensues and there is little that the women can do to stop it unless they are able to assert themselves. Some midwives find themselves unable to halt the medical intervention and less able to be an advocate for the women in their care. Strangely, as long as women stay at home to labour, their length of labour will not be recorded officially, and they will maximise their chance of delivering their baby normally. Moreover, women tend to potter about in the house while in labour and automatically assume an upright position, again maximising their chance of a normal delivery.

Slade et al (1993) compared women's experiences and expectations of antenatal preparations and found that women expected to exert more control over their pain by use of their coping methods than actually occurred. Slade (1996) suggests that many women may not translate preparation into practice. One theory is that during antenatal education, women may be given too much information or the information may be too generalised. This may account for the women's inability to translate the large amount of information given to them into practical coping strategies during labour.

Wide variation in content of antenatal classes and attendance

There appears to be wide variation in the content and structure of antenatal classes within maternity units, local authorities, health centres and private consumer bodies, such as the National Childbirth Trust. The variation also includes differences in the value of classes or sessions, timing and allocation of resources regarding the provision of antenatal education (Murphy-Black, 1990, 1991; Tew, 1990; Slade, 1996). This may explain why attendance at antenatal education ranged from 81%, based on those who attended at least one session (Michie et al, 1992), to as low as 20% in some health authorities (Byrne-Lynch, 1991; Slade, 1996; Cliff and Deery, 1997; Lee and Shorten, 1999).

Attendance at antenatal classes has never reached the numbers that midwives would like to attain. In a national study with a large representative sample, Jacoby (1988) found that only 41% of women attended classes. The majority of these were white caucasian women from non-manual social classes having their first baby. In addition, many of these women did not attend the full course.

In another study, Bennett et al (1985) found that frequent attendees were older. Michie et al (1992) found significant differences in the social classes of attendees, with more women from social classes I and II (professional groups) attending than from classes III and IV (working classes).

In another review (Tew, 1990), participation in classes ranged from 18% in the 1970s to 34% in 1985. Indeed, the question of poor attendance at antenatal classes cannot be ignored. Attendance at antenatal classes today remains much the same two decades later, although the style and content of education has changed over the years to reflect cultural needs and social attitudes (Combes and Schonveld, 1992; Schott and Henley, 1996; Slade, 1996). Some parent education classes address individual learning needs and have moved towards a more adult-centred learning style (Schott and Henley, 1996). A recent study in Italy found that only 23% of women attended classes, and these were mostly women without previous children, who had a higher level of education and were office workers (Spinelli et al, 2003).

Several authors have identified the need to restructure the way that parent education is provided (Murphy-Black, 1990; Schott and Henley, 1996; Nolan and Hicks, 1997; Lee and Shorten, 1999; Jansen and Blizzard, 1999; Nolan, 1999) as a means of addressing falling attendance. Ideas range from changing the timing and venue of classes, considering whether the session should be given in groups, in pairs, and with or without partner involvement, to the importance of ice-breaker sessions and asking women what they want at the start of the session.

Other studies stress the importance of providing adequate information and challenge the teaching and the educator to be flexible and to improve on traditional education classes to meet the needs of modern women (Robertson, 1994; Rees, 1996; Nolan, 1998; Behnke, 2000). How much of the information is retained and applied to women in their decision-making during labour is largely unknown. It is argued that women cannot be expected to make quality decisions and explicit choices pertinent to their individual needs and preferences during their pregnancy or labour if they are uninformed about the options available to them (Oliver et al, 1996; Oakley, 1980; Coppen, 2002). Robertson (1999) suggested that antenatal education has never been evaluated seriously, and Handfield (1997) highlighted the need for a randomised controlled trial to evaluate the effectiveness of antenatal education.

Benefits of knowledge gained at antenatal classes

To what extent are antenatal preparation classes beneficial to women? Hillier and Slade (1989) assessed women's knowledge levels at the start of the antenatal classes and after the final class, and found a significant increase in knowledge after the classes. How knowledge was assessed was not clear and there was no control group as the women were self-selected. Although the study identified the benefits of antenatal classes on the women's knowledge bases, it did not indicate whether the knowledge gained influenced factors such as choice, decision-making, birth outcome and satisfaction levels before or during labour. Antenatal classes are not the only method of providing education to pregnant women: women may gain their knowledge of labour and receive information from their midwives during antenatal check-ups, through the media, from friends and relatives, and through reading books and magazines. Women can also learn from their own experiences of labour.

An American study (Allen and Ries, 1985) found that antenatal education about the health effects of smoking and alcohol consumption was effective in increasing women's knowledge and achieving behavioural change in a group of women.

A population-based observation study in Italy (Spinelli et al, 2003) found that women who attended antenatal classes appeared to improve their knowledge and competence and gained greater satisfaction from the childbirth experience.

A study in Australia (Rolls and Cutts, 2001) compared the effectiveness of a traditional system of education with that of a new approach to educating women. The study was based on a prospective, longitudinal, pre-test/post-test experimental design: 70 first-time pregnant women and their partners were recruited to an educational programme designed to support and educate women about their expectations of labour and address the postnatal fears of expectant parents. Findings showed that there was increased knowledge of pregnancy, labour, birth and the postnatal period among the experimental group in pre- to midway assessments. However, there were no differences between the groups in the overall mean across assessments, and attendance at antenatal education was found not to be associated with a positive experience of going home with a new baby among first-time mothers.

In a Cochrane review to assess the effects of antenatal education on knowledge acquisition and psychosocial factors in labour, Gagnon (2001) found only six trials, involving a total of 1443 women. The largest of the studies, involving 1275 women, was found to be of high quality. It examined an educational intervention to increase the rate of vaginal birth after caesarean section. The review concluded that the effects of general antenatal education remain unknown, and that individualised prenatal education aimed at avoiding caesarean birth was of little value as the results showed that it did not increase the rate of vaginal birth after caesarean section. How the educational intervention was given or what information was disseminated was not elaborated. The quality of the methodology of the remaining five studies was uncertain as attrition rates and methods of randomisation were not clear. The true effects of antenatal education on the women's knowledge and ability to make decisions concerning the use of different positions in labour remain largely unknown.

Summary

Overall, little is known about the quality of the information provided in antenatal classes. Whether antenatal preparation leads to beneficial outcomes is a complex question, since it involves defining what constitutes a beneficial outcome and for whom (Slade, 1996). Good quality studies on the benefits or effects of antenatal education on knowledge acquisition, sense of control or labour outcomes were limited (Gagnon, 2001).

Many studies on antenatal preparation assessed its impact on physical and psychosocial outcomes (Timm, 1979; Oakley, 1980; Allen and Ries, 1985; Simkin and Enkin, 1989; Gagnon, 2001). Others concentrated on the benefits of an educational programme as a whole (Murphy-Black, 1990; Schott and Henley, 1996; Slade, 1996; Nolan, 1999; Rolls and Cutts, 2001). However, many of these studies were descriptive, discussed the basis of antenatal education as a whole, and did not compare the effects of different educational strategies. Even less is known about women's views on the choices of birthing positions available to them in labour, or to what extent parent education influences a woman's decision-making process.

In this book, the results of research undertaken by the author to assess the effectiveness of focused information on women's knowledge levels, and whether being informed significantly increases women's decisions to use upright positions for labour and childbirth, will be discussed. This research will thus provide evidence on whether there is an expressed need for women to be informed of the various birthing positions in order to make an educated and informed decision.

The main aim of the investigation was to ascertain whether the provision of 'focused' information, as opposed to 'general' information, was superior in terms of knowledge gained, satisfaction, reduced decisional conflict and improved decision-making. A second aim was to test the hypothesis that the provision of focused information will enhance knowledge, reduce decisional conflict and empower women to take control of their decision-making in childbirth.

A systematic review of the literature on the use of different birthing positions, including women's and midwives' views, was undertaken before the trial. The review identified gaps in the literature on the benefits and use of upright birthing positions and on women's decision-making processes, including the role of midwives.

A survey to investigate the views and attitudes of midwives towards the use of alternative positions in labour and delivery will also be reported in Section II of this book.

A double-blind randomised controlled trial was considered the most appropriate methodology for a study to compare the effects of the provision of focused information (the intervention) *vs* general information on women's decision-making during labour and childbirth. To ease the decision-making process and to enable measurement of the degree of women's preference for one position over another, a new decision instrument, entitled a decision analysis preference triage (ADAPT; *Appendix 1*), was developed for the trial. All the women in the trial completed ADAPT before and after the educational session, and the findings were compared to determine women's decisions and preferences regarding their choice of birthing positions. The results will show what women want – from their midwives and for themselves – once they are informed of their options regarding their choice of birthing positions.

CHAPTER 3

Historical perspective and the medicalisation of birthing positions

To understand the rationale for the use of recumbent positions in clinical practice today, we need to look at the history of birthing positions, particularly the events that led to the hospitalisation of all women in labour by politicians, and the 'medicalisation of childbirth' that followed the introduction of birth technology and the influence of obstetricians in the birthplace. This chapter highlights the anthropological and historical perspectives of childbirth positions and discusses the medicalisation of birthing positions by obstetricians and midwives.

Anthropological and historical perspectives of birthing positions

The semi-recumbent, dorsal and lithotomy positions seem to be used routinely in hospitals in contemporary Western society today (Inch, 1982b; Thomson, 1988; Thomson, 1995; Coppen, 1997). Yet the routine use of such positions is rarely found in anthropological or historical studies (Rigby, 1857; Englemann, 1882; Jarcho, 1929; Hewes, 1957; Dening, 1982; Russell, 1982; Klein-Tebbe et al, 1996; Gupta and Nikodem, 2000b). The way we sit, stand, kneel or squat is determined not only by human anatomy but also by culture. According to Hewes (1957), the human body is capable of assuming something in the order of 1000 different steady postures (steady being defined as a static position that can be maintained comfortably for some time). Yet during childbirth, only a limited number of positions have been used over the centuries, notably the recumbent and chair-sitting postures used by Westerners, and the upright positions of squatting, standing and crouching favoured by Asiatic and Eastern populations (Jarcho, 1929; Hewes, 1957; Dening 1982; Russell, 1982).

The place of furniture in childbirth

Chair sitting and furniture, possibly the chief distinguishing postural attributes of Western civilisation, go hand in hand, according to Hewes (1957). But which came first – the invention of birthing stools and chairs or the desire to maintain the upright position in labour – is more difficult to identify. Stools and chairs were used in Egypt and Mesopotamia at least 5000 years ago, and by the Chinese, Japanese and Koreans only 3000 years ago. Even today, many people would choose to sit comfortably on the floor for family meals, resting, reading or sewing, rather than on a stool or chair, as it is culturally acceptable.

More widely practised than chair sitting is the deep squat, used for cooking over a low, hot stone fire, for resting and for ablutions. To the Western world, this may seem an undignified and highly primitive posture; indeed, Reynolds (1991) referred to the standing and squatting postures as primitive. Interestingly, however, he found that women and their partners preferred these positions for birthing. Furthermore, millions of people in many parts of Asia, Africa, Latin America and Oceania customarily work and rest in the squatting position (Engelmann, 1882; Hewes, 1957; Naroll et al, 1961).

Russell (1982) reported the use of birth stools in Greece and Egypt. Fasbender (1906) claimed that the first account of a birthing stool in history occurred in the work of Soranus of Ephesus in the 2nd Century AD. However, a much earlier account of the use of birthing stools was given in the Old Testament Book of Exodus (*New King James Bible*, 2000; *The Holy Bible* (NIV), 2004) before the birth of Christ. To quote the King of Egypt addressing the Hebrew midwives:

> '*And he said, When ye do the office of a midwife to the Hebrew women, and see them upon the stools...*'

Exodus 1:16

The use of birth stools in Egypt was documented in several medical papyri (Mayer, 1942) and was represented in stone reliefs in the Birth House at Luxor around 1450 BC (Weindler, 1915). Among the Greeks, Hippocrates, a midwife's son (De Lee, 1934), recommended the obstetric chair (Thompson, 1957). At that time, women were usually confined semi-recumbent in bed (Diepgen, 1937; Inch, 1982a), except in difficult cases, when the obstetric chair was used (Housholder, 1974).

Cultural positions in labour

Engelmann (1882), in his anthropological study of normal labour in primitive societies, encompassing 54 countries from all continents, found that certain tribes and races used traditional birthing positions such as squatting, kneeling, sitting, standing, and the suspended position held by ropes or thick cloths swung over large tree trunks. Horizontal positions such as supine, prone and dorsal were used more by Western societies. Engelmann found that women would choose several positions during the course of labour. However, during the second stage of labour, upright positions were used more by all women, with horizontal positions rarely being used.

Jarcho (1934) concurred with Engelmann's findings, describing how adept women were at maintaining the upright posture in childbirth. In another study, Jarcho (1929) observed that Indian women adopted the crouching position with one knee flexed completely on the ground and the other knee raised to deliver their babies. The rationale for this position is evident from the following quote by Jarcho (1929, p.257):

'If the fetal head is displaced into one of the iliac fossae, it may be forced back over the inlet if the knee on the side of the displacement is raised.'

The squatting position was also clearly described by Jarcho (1929), who observed that among the Indian tribes the Tonkawa women maintained the squatting posture (*Figure 1.5*, p.8) or semi-squatting posture (*Figures 1.6a & b*, p.8) until after expulsion of the child. *Figure 1.7* (p.9) shows a woman delivering or labouring with the aid of a rope. According to Chinese custom, the squatting posture favours the delivery of the baby, separation of the placenta and involution of the uterus (Jarcho, 1929; Russell, 1982).

Atwood (1976) provided further anthropological and historical insights into the use of different positions in labour and childbirth. He found that four distinct upright positions – the standing, sitting, squatting and kneeling positions – have been used in non-Western cultures, whereas neutral positions, such as the lithotomy, head-down, hanging leg, lateral prone, lateral, prone, semi-recumbent and knee and elbow positions, were used in Western cultures. An interaction between the physical and cultural aspects of childbirth is therefore apparent from his findings. Atwood's study also provided further insight into the cross-cultural study by Ford (1945) of women from 39 primitive societies. Ford found that 16 societies used the sitting position, 11 the kneeling position, two the squatting position and 10 some form of alternative position.

Another extensive study was conducted by Naroll et al (1961) on first-hand reports recorded in the Human Relations Area Files, from which it was possible to collect statistics on a large sample of human societies from all over the world. Naroll et al collected and tabulated data on the use of upright positions by 76 primitive tribes from Asia, Africa, Oceania and the Americas. They found that of the 76 primitive (tribal) cultures studied, 62 used an upright position (21 the kneeling position, 15 the squatting position, 5 the standing position and 19 the all-fours position – two files were unaccounted for). In the other 14 tribes, most births occurred in neutral positions, such as the supine, prone or all-fours position. It is interesting that the all-fours position was categorised as a neutral position, and not an upright or alternative position as it is better known today.

Birthing position: instinct vs custom

An instinctive preference for the squatting position has also been documented in studies on labour in primitive women (Rigby, 1857; Engelmann, 1882; Ford, 1945). However, where instinct ended and custom began is less clear. According to Housholder (1974), the primate squatting position was for the most part retained among primitive people. What did Housholder mean by primitive people? Was he referring to the uneducated and unenlightened individuals who adopted what would appear to be a natural position for them, or was he referring to the population of the non-Western world as a whole? Current practice suggests that some Western women would be happy to use the squatting position, which has been found to significantly reduce the length of labour, improve perineal integrity and reduce the risk of shoulder dystocia (Golay et al, 1993).

Rigby was an author ahead of his time. An eminent obstetrician, he posed the question in his research (Rigby, 1857): 'What is the natural position of a woman in labour?' From his observation of 100 women in labour, Rigby found that, without any antenatal preparation, free from Western influences and left to their own devices, most women would labour in the upright position. Significantly, the majority of the women (82%) assumed the upright position for delivery. Of these, 44% adopted the standing position, 34% the squatting or crouching positions and 4% the kneeling position.

It is sobering to note that more than a century ago, writers such as Lusk (1894) and Rigby (1857) suggested that women should be left to labour on their own and choose a posture that was suited to their individual needs and volition without interference from professionals – a point well made. I am all for giving women every opportunity to labour without interference and unnecessary intervention. I believe that most women are quite capable of delivering normally – they just have to believe in themselves and, most importantly, optimise their chance of successful labour by keeping mobile, avoiding epidural analgesia and adopting the upright position throughout labour.

Figure 3.1 shows some suggested upright positions that women may wish

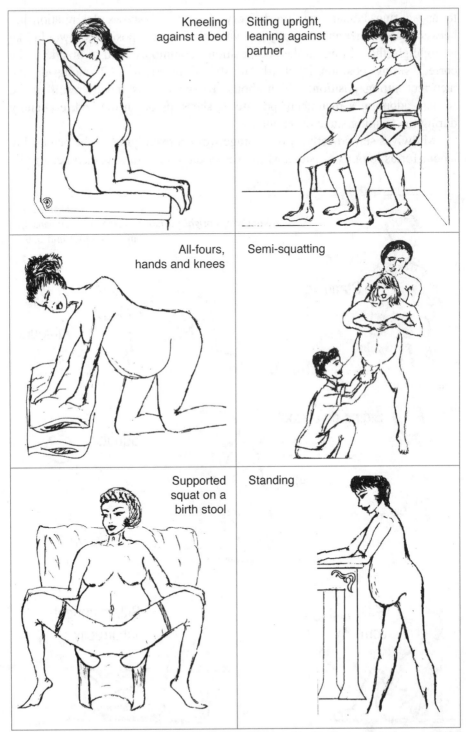

Figure 3.1:A variety of upright birthing positions. (Illustrated by Liz Seah and R Coppen, 2002)

to use during labour and for delivery. *Figure 3.2* shows the relationship between the mother and the baby in a variety of upright positions. I would like to highlight the 'sitting on the bed position', commonly used in practice. The correct sitting position is clearly illustrated in *Figure 3.2*, alongside the incorrect sitting position, which should be avoided as it will result in the woman adopting a recumbent posture as she slips down the bed, especially during the pushing stage of labour.

Midwives should actively discourage women from lying on the bed during labour for as long as possible. Midwives often tell me that women need to lie

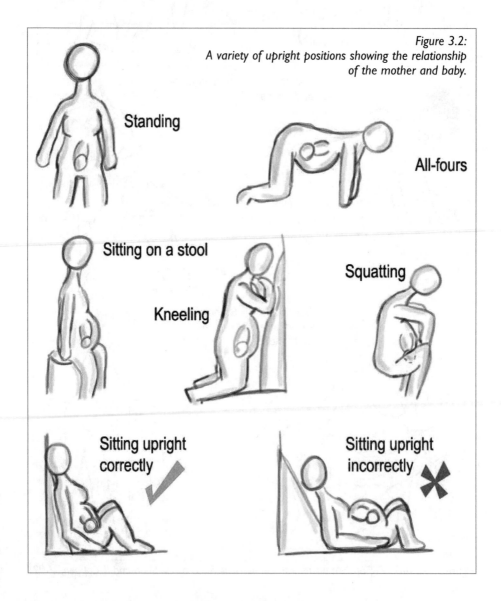

Figure 3.2:
A variety of upright positions showing the relationship of the mother and baby.

Standing

All-fours

Sitting on a stool

Kneeling

Squatting

Sitting upright correctly

Sitting upright incorrectly

on the bed during labour because they are tired and exhausted. I would argue that, on the contrary, it is important to appreciate that the term 'to labour' means 'to work, to toil, to sweat, to strive and [my favourite] to endeavour' (Soanes, 2000). Midwives are acutely aware that women in labour go through several hours of hard work. They have a professional duty of care to forewarn women that it is going to be a tiring, exhausting experience, but it is time limited. My advice to all women in labour is: 'Don't give up, actively move around and press on! There will be much joy when the baby is born, your efforts will not be in vain and you will very soon forget the pain'. It never ceases to amaze me how quickly women forget the pain once the baby is born. I often rue the day the bed was invented for women to lie on in labour. It has done them no favours.

Birthing in bed first established itself among the middle and upper classes towards the mid-18th century with the advent of 'man-midwives' (now known as obstetricians) (Graham, 1960). Shorter (1991) also commented that doctors preferred women to lie on their backs (recumbent position) during labour and delivery because it was convenient and they thought it might help the women to rest. By all means use the bed for resting between contractions, to lie on for a short time, or to take a 'mini-rest' of no more than 15 minutes at a time to regain your strength and energy, but never lie on the bed for any length of time, as there is clear evidence that this will delay the progress of labour and may decrease the strength of contractions and heighten labour pains.

A variety of birth aids are available in most maternity units, which women can use freely during labour. *Figure 3.3a* shows a woman sitting on a birth ball, holding on to a long braid, which she can grab or pull downwards during contractions to ease labour pains. In some maternity units, the top of the braid is secured firmly to the ceiling (*Figure 3.3b*). *Figure 3.3b* also shows a wooden birth stool, which women can use to help them maintain an upright posture in labour and cope with the pain. A midwife can be seen demonstrating the use of a birth stool in *Figure 3.3c*, and *Figure 3.3d* shows a luxurious birth pool for waterbirth and relaxation seen in an exhibition in Vienna. It is interesting to note that birth chairs and stools were already in use more than 100 years ago (*Figure 3.4*).

A Latin-American collaborative study (Caldeyro-Barcia, 1979a, 1979b; Schwarcz et al, 1977) involving 11 maternity hospitals in seven countries found that only 5% of women elected to lie down in bed and 95% preferred to walk, stand or sit upright during labour. Roberts et al (1983) found that women preferred to stand during labour as they found it more comfortable and less painful than lying on the bed. Yet in current practice, most women in labour lie on the bed most of the time. Why is this so? Is it because they have not been encouraged to walk around or, worse, that they have been advised to do so by midwives and healthcare professionals, or that they are none the wiser for knowing what is best for them?

Influence of Western cultures on birth positions

Historical evidence suggests that throughout the world in Western and non-Western societies, vertical positions were the most prevalent way to give birth until the 18th century (Engelmann, 1882; Inch, 1982b; Poschl, 1987; Limburg and Smulders, 1992). Birth scenes from early Virginia, USA, in the treatise by Englemann (1882), demonstrate the compromise between the accoucheur who

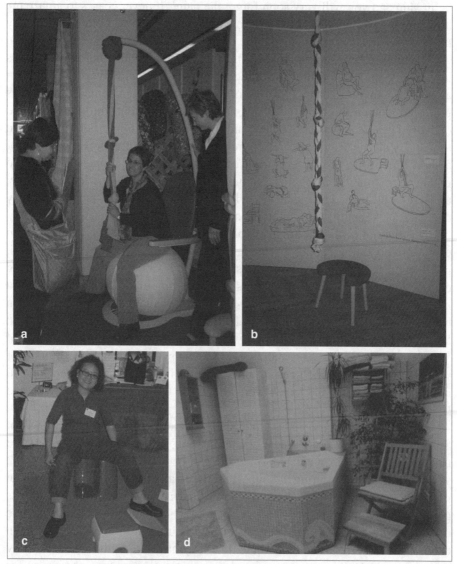

Figure 3.3: A variety of modern birthing aids: (a) birth ball and braid; (b) birth rope and wooden stool; (c) demonstration of the use of a birth stool; (d) birth pool.

Figure 3.4:
Victorian birth
chairs and stools.

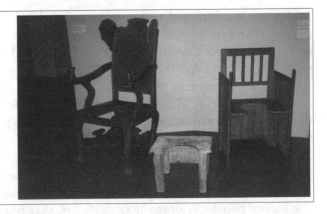

wanted to get to the perineum and the woman who wanted to squat. Such a compromise today would often mean that the midwife would either actively encourage the woman to squat or kneel or stand, or cajole the woman to turn onto her back to allow the midwife access to the perineum.

Western influences on traditional practices were also apparent in Hillier's (2003) accounts of women's stories of their childbirth experience. In one account a midwife trained in Western practices working in Ghana instructed a woman in the second stage of labour to assume a lying down position. The woman was apparently satisfied with this as she too had been influenced to think that squatting was for the peasants and the uneducated. In contrast, another midwife actively encouraged a woman to adopt the kneeling position for delivery; however, this woman and the midwife were both from the Amish community, who are not easily influenced by the Western world. This suggests that without Western influences, midwives would be free to use their instinctive skills and would deliver women in the upright posture.

In the 15th century, the development of birthing aids meant that midwives in Germany began to use the birthing stool, adopting the idea from Italy where such stools had been used for centuries (Inch, 1982b; Shorter, 1991). By the 16th century, birthing stools were in common use in the cities of central Europe (Martin, 1917). In the 18th century, Henrik van Deventer, a Dutch obstetrician who later became known as the 'father of modern midwifery', described the use of an obstetric chair for delivery in 1701 (Alaily, 1996; Garrison, 1929). He developed an obstetric stool that resembled a backless chair with an opening in the seat of the chair; he claimed that with this chair, the coccyx would be free and thus able to move out of the way of the descending head. The back could move freely so the woman could adopt any position she wished. With this newly designed chair, women were able to move more easily from the supported squat of the birthing stool to a kneeling or all-fours position. This obstetric stool was chosen as an apparatus for the proper positioning of the woman in labour. It can be viewed as an adaptation of the squatting position (Housholder, 1974).

By the late 18th and 19th centuries, the obstetric chair had become very popular in Germany, especially among wealthy women, probably more for the quality of the stool than its practicality as stools and chairs then were made of expensive material and very heavy (Alaily, 1996). Also, the French physician Ambrose Paré recommended the use of the birthing chair, and the French obstetrician François Mauriceau described a chair for delivery (Alaily, 1996). European and American chairs were designed during the 18th century, and birth stools or chairs for delivering women are still in use today.

The popularity of the birthing chair in the UK, however, has waned over the years, compared with its Dutch counterpart, the Birth-Mate stool from Amsterdam, which is still in common use today (Limburg and Smulders, 1992). The lack of popularity of the stool in the UK may be due to the adverse effects found in several studies, such as increased blood loss and perineal trauma (Cottrell and Shannahan, 1986; Turner et al, 1986; Stewart and Spiby, 1989a). Their high cost, ranging from £250 to £4000 per chair, may also contribute to their lack of popularity (Alaily, 1996). A Berlin doctor (Stucky, 1965) claimed that 'stools made delivery harder rather than easier'; however, it has since been argued that this was because the old stools were harder and more uncomfortable than stools today (Shorter, 1991), which are made of firm plastic or solid wood with a smooth curvature, and are ergonomically designed.

With the decline in use of the birthing stool, women may have no choice but to use the bed during labour. Indeed, by the mid-to-late 18th century, Mauriceau appeared to have changed his views about upright posture and recommended the semi-recumbent position for delivery on the bed, believing that it would be more comfortable for the mother (Alaily, 1996). It was also evident that 'man midwives' preferred women to lie on their side with their backs facing away from the physician. The bed therefore became established practice among the middle and upper classes around the mid-18th century (Shorter, 1991). In 1844, Rigby argued that doctors had been using this position for over a century, with some preferring mothers to deliver on their backs (Leishman, 1879).

Anthropological and historical evidence therefore suggests that most women in the non-Westernised world commonly used upright positions for labour and childbirth. The instinctive use of the squatting position, as a culturally accepted position adopted by Eastern, African and Asiatic women, cannot be ignored. Cultural differences leading to the adoption of different positions have been examined. Western influences led to the use of furniture, e.g. the chair, bench or stool, to aid delivery and provide a more dignified position, while still enabling women to maintain the upright position. Decline in the use of the birthing stool or chair over the past decade may be due to known adverse effects, personal preference, male dominance in childbirth practices, or high cost. Current practice is seeing a resurgence in use of the birthing stool; however, this is more common in birthing centres than maternity units, unless the midwife is confident in its use.

The 'medicalisation' of birthing positions

To understand the reasons for the continued use of recumbent positions in childbirth today, it is important to look at the influence of doctors, birth attendants (midwives) and medical technology. Factors contributing to the 'medicalisation' of birthing positions, including the move from home to hospital births, will be discussed.

The practice of obstetrics and the management of women in labour have been in the hands of midwives for centuries while the majority of births took place at home (Fields et al, 1965; Oakley, 1980; Campbell and MacFarlane, 1986, 1990; Tew, 1990).

Before the routine admission of women to hospitals, obstetricians in the UK played a minor role in the care of women in labour. Antenatal care was in the hands of midwives, as was the total care of women in labour (these were mostly home births by midwives) and during the postnatal period. Doctors were only called upon when complications arose and only then were women admitted to the hospital. Interventions by obstetricians, e.g. for induction of labour, made its appearance when obstetrics became a part of medical science (Fields et al, 1965; Inch, 1982a).

Slowly, but inevitably, obstetricians became increasingly influential within the childbirth domain, as noted in a midwifery textbook as early as 1908 (Tew, 1990). Soon the midwife, once a central figure in a woman's labour, became secondary to the obstetrician – so much so that many midwives today feel that they lack the confidence to provide the kind of intervention-free care that was previously considered the norm. For example, midwives were 'instructed' by doctors to manage delivery by allowing the women to move around as they wished, but only in the first stage of labour, and then to 'put women to bed' in the second stage of labour (Inch, 1982b; Towler and Bramall, 1986). Yet it is in this crucial stage of labour that women must be encouraged to maintain the upright position. Indeed, misguided midwives were instructed that it would help women to push more effectively if the woman's leg was raised onto stirrups in the lithotomy position on the bed (Towler and Bramall, 1986). It was said that such a position was convenient for the birth attendant, and made it easy to monitor the baby's heart rate and repair episiotomies (Hillier, 2003). Such instructions became the norm as midwives inadvertently prevented women from choosing to deliver in the upright position, and may thus have unknowingly delayed women's progress in labour (Tew, 1990; Coppen, 1997). Even today, many obstetricians and some midwives are still delivering women in the lithotomy position despite evidence contraindicating its use (Hillier, 2003).

The concept of giving women choice or control in childbirth began to diminish as obstetricians took on a higher profile in the care of pregnant women. In addition, the introduction of the National Health Service for all, in the UK in 1948, provided the impetus for the move from the home to the hospital environment, and established the obstetrician as a central and dominant figure in the care of the woman during childbirth (Symonds and Hunt, 1996; Tew, 1990; Garcia et al, 1990). Many midwives today, especially in America, are having to defend their right to practise 'active birth' and 'natural childbirth', as they strive to be advocates for women while hospital privileges are denied them and home birth is still highly controversial (Hillier, 2003).

The decision to hospitalise all women in labour was influenced by high levels of maternal mortality in the 1930s and the belief that hospital birth was safer than home birth (Inch, 1982a; Tew, 1990; Symonds and Hunt, 1996; Madi, 2000). The move from a home to a hospital birth had less to do with meeting the needs of women and more to do with the preoccupation with safety during childbirth. It has been mooted that such a major change in health policy was not based on any evidence that home births were unsafe (Kitzinger and Davis, 1978, Tew 1990). The Peel Report (Standing Maternity and Midwifery Advisory Committee, 1970) played a significant role in the total move from the then 12.4% home-birth rate to 100% hospital births. The chairman Sir Robert Peel claimed that it would be safer for women to deliver in a hospital environment and went on to recommend 100% hospital deliveries. The move from home to hospital also meant that the way women delivered their baby changed, since the bed is a central focus in all hospital births. This in turn led to restrictions in the choice of birthing positions for women (Tew, 1990; Shorter, 1991).

In contrast, women were not restricted to the bed at home, and many women could choose to give birth in upright positions, such as standing or kneeling (Bastian, 1994; Coppen, 1997). Other favourable positions, such as the all-fours position, standing, and sitting on a birthing stool have been reported to assist in labour considerably, especially when the baby is lying in the posterior position (Biancuzzo, 1991; Bastian, 1994; Henty, 1998). Bruner et al (1998) highlighted the benefit of the all-fours position in managing shoulder dystocia. Although many deliveries were conducted on the bed at home, the main difference between home birth and hospital birth was that women were able to exercise their personal choice more effectively with regard to birthing positions in labour and childbirth (Bastian, 1994; Coppen, 1997; Henty, 1998).

As more and more women in the UK delivered in hospital, there was a rise in intervention rates, and instrumental delivery and caesarean section became an all too familiar pattern in many maternity units (Inch, 1982a; Oakley, 1980, 1986, Tew, 1990; Shorter, 1991). These events have been termed a 'cascade of intervention' (MacLennan, 1978; Inch, 1982a) or an 'orgy of intervention' (Shorter, 1991), done in the name of 'safety for the fetus'. Yet many of these interventions have not been properly evaluated in clinical practice, and until recently were not questioned. Oakley (1980) first took up the challenge to de-medicalise childbirth by calling on all health professionals to address the rising tide of unnecessary medical interventions, e.g. induction of labour with oxytocics, forceps deliveries and episiotomies.

Oakley (1980) went on to describe how easy it was for women to be influenced by such technology and interventions under the pretext that it would provide a better outcome or better satisfaction. Terms such as 'medicalisation of childbirth', 'medicalisation of life', 'medicalisation of reproduction' and 'medicalisation of pregnancy' have all been used (Oakley, 1980, 1986) synonymously to mean a form of 'interference' with human nature, in this case the natural process of birth, life, reproduction and pregnancy. In clinical practice today, 'medicalisation of childbirth' has come to signify institutionalisation, i.e. birth in a hospital environment within a clinical setting, surrounded by increasing technology, e.g. epidural analgesia and routine fetal monitoring, interventions such as episiotomy and artificial rupture of the membranes (ARM) with an implement such as the 'kockers' or hook, and the inherent rules and routines of hospital practice (Paciornik, 1980; Kitzinger and Walters, 1981, 1988; Moore, 1997).

As the number of interventions rose, so the midwife's role became eroded as obstetricians took over almost all the maternity care of women (Inch, 1982a; Tew, 1990; Shorter, 1991; Oakley and Richards, 1990). Wendy Savage, an obstetrician, pointed out that in the 20th century the power of the obstetrician rose to unprecedented heights (Savage, 1986). Savage questioned the rise in obstetric intervention and highlighted the need to base practice more on scientific evidence and less on the established norm. Further examples of doctors interfering with childbirth can be seen in studies where doctors advocated the use of the bed for delivery and the use of recumbent positions to help women in labour (Inch, 1982b; Towler and Brammall ,1986; Tew, 1990; Shorter, 1991; Alaily, 1996). Professionals at the time hardly questioned the recommendation that women should be delivering in the recumbent or supine position, despite evidence that the upright position is physiologically more efficient in assisting the descent of the fetus (Tew, 1990; De Jong et al, 1997; De Jonge et al, 2004) and improving fetal oxygenation (Aldrich et al, 1995).

It was not until later that midwives began to express concern over the erosion of their role as advocates of women-centred care (Campbell and MacFarlane, 1990; Tew, 1990). Michel Odent, a French obstetrician, is a proponent of a non-interventionist approach to childbirth; his philosophy is that labour should be left undisturbed and women should be encouraged to adopt the position that suits them best (Odent, 1984).

Hence the 'medicalisation of birthing positions', and therefore the routine use of recumbent positions, occurred at the same time as the move from hospital to home birth, and medical intervention became the norm in many hospitals in the UK. This was evident as women began to rebel against the regimentation of birth and demanded far greater choice of postures such as standing, kneeling or squatting (Tew, 1990).

In response to this demand, obstetricians invested in birth chairs and bean-bags, although monitoring of women in labour continued to have high priority (Tew, 1990). Interestingly, a controversial study by a group of obstetricians (Burger et al, 1996) advocated the possibility and benefits of using birthing chairs for breech delivery. The use of birth chairs was popular in the 1970s and 80s, as numerous studies have shown (Calder et al, 1983; Cottrell and Shannahan, 1986, 1987; Crowley et al, 1991; Stewart et al, 1983; Stewart and Spiby, 1989a; Turner, 1986; Waldenstrom and Gottval, 1991).

Oakley (1980) argued that doctors must come to terms with the fact that childbearing is a natural and normal event, and that all over the industrialised world 97% of the female population is capable of delivering babies safely and without complications. Kloosterman (1975) was certain that 80–90% of women were perfectly capable of delivering themselves normally without help, and presumably in whatever position they chose. He added:

> *'Spontaneous labour in a healthy woman is an event marked by a number of processes which are so complex, so perfectly attuned to each other that any interference will only detract from their optimal character...'*

> (Kloosterman, 1975, p.287)

Tew (1990) also pointed out that when a woman adopts a recumbent position it implies weakness, inferiority and submission to the superiority of the obstetrician. In my experience I have also noted that when women are lying in bed they have to 'look up' to the midwives and obstetricians when communicating with them, as they stand by their bedside, whereas the reverse is true when women adopt the upright position. For example, midwives would spontaneously assume a lower position when talking to women in a kneeling, squatting or all-fours position. Few would find it difficult to communicate effectively otherwise. The continued use of recumbent positions is compounded by the fact that doctors who worked and taught in hospitals enforced recumbence and it eventually became accepted as the normal birth position by midwives (Tew, 1990). Sheila Kitzinger (1981, 1983), a proponent of natural childbirth, and Wendy Savage (1986), an obstetrician, spoke up for women's rights. They played an active part in encouraging women to stand up for their rights and refuse unnecessary interventions by health professionals.

At the same time, societies such as the National Childbirth Trust and Action for the Improvement of Maternity Services called for the return of women-centred care. Several high-profile government reports have since been published, which identified the need to redress the problems of unnecessary intervention and advocated attention to the needs of the mother. The three Cs – Choice, Control and Continuity of care – were first highlighted by the Maternity Services Advisory Committee (1982, 1984, 1985). Three reports entitled *Maternity Care in Action* heralded the importance of humanising the maternity care services. They promoted the need to provide women with choice and control during the antenatal, intrapartum and postpartum period. Unfortunately, these reports did not do much to stem the rising rate of intervention, although they did provide a platform for midwives to discuss changes in pregnancy care.

It was not until publication of the Winterton Report by the House of Commons Health Select Committee (1992) that women were given more control over the decision-making process. At last, women's needs were being taken more seriously, as women began to state their preferred choice of care and identify what they really wanted from the maternity services. Important issues, such as the place of delivery, women having more control over their body and more choices of care delivery, were just some of the points raised from this report.

Unfortunately, high-profile reports such as those from the Maternity Services Advisory Committee (1982, 1984, 1985) and the Winterton Report have done little to change some of the old practices, such as early admission in labour, continuous electronic fetal monitoring and the use of recumbent positions, to name a few.

A survey of women's views of maternity care in mid-Surrey showed that the majority of the women (75%) delivered in the semi-recumbent position and 11% in the recumbent position. Yet a quarter of the women said that, given the choice, they would have chosen the upright position (Coppen, 1994). In a review of the literature on management of the second stage of labour, Thomson (1988) questioned current UK policies that required women to deliver in the semi-recumbent dorsal position. She demonstrated logically that the woman is likely to slip down the bed and therefore lose any of the theoretical advantage of gravity, and that the sacrum is fixed when the woman lies on her back. Consequently, women would be unable to take advantage of any potential outward movement, which may increase the size of the pelvis (Thomson, 1988).

In the industrialised world today, labour is seen not as a physiological and normal event best managed by leaving well alone, but as a pathological event to be managed and interfered with to ensure a safe delivery. In clinical practice, when women are admitted in labour it is not uncommon to see them being confined to bed, monitored continuously for no reason other than it is hospital protocol, and have decisions about their care made for them. Savage (1986) added that doctors themselves lack adequate information and should not be the primary decision-maker in the care of women in labour. Indeed, I would suggest that a joint tripartite process, where women partake in the decision-making together with their midwife and doctor, should be the way forward.

However, it has taken another government report *A First Class Service* (Department of Health, 1998b), which called for the setting up of clinical governance and the National Institute for Clinical Excellence (NICE), for professionals to take stock and address the problems of providing unnecessary intervention without clear evidence. This report pointed out that clinical decisions should only be made when based on the best available evidence (Dobson, 1998; NICE, 2003). Interestingly, Savage (1986) made the same statement more than a decade ago.

Since the publication of this report, attempts have been made to change the unfavourable practice of continuous fetal monitoring for all women in labour. The purpose of this is to ensure that only women who are at risk are monitored, as there is no evidence that electronic fetal monitoring has any benefits for low-risk women (WHO, 1999; NICE, 2001). A report from NICE (2003) set out clear guidelines and evidence-based information on the use of electronic fetal monitoring. It stated clearly that assessment of fetal wellbeing is only one component of intrapartum care and that due consideration must be given to maternal preference. It also added:

'A balance must be struck between the objective of maximising the detection of problems in the baby and that of minimising the number of unnecessary maternal interventions.'

(NICE, 2003, p.3)

Unfortunately, it would appear that not enough is being done to stem the use of continuous fetal monitoring. I was dismayed to hear from a medical colleague recently that one of the reasons why continuous monitoring is still used in practice today is that the NICE report is seen only as a 'guideline' to good practice and not necessarily something to be followed! I would argue that unnecessary fetal monitoring is a form of intervention that compels women to lie in bed most of the time. This would in turn prevent, discourage and deter women from maintaining the upright position during labour, which would in turn lead to a 'cascade of intervention' if labour did not progress according to the doctor's preference or unit protocol.

To end on a positive note, the interventionist approach to childbirth care, the 'medicalisation of childbirth' and the 'medicalisation of birthing positions' may indeed be coming to an end, as obstetricians and midwives in this country take stock of the government's most recent health document, the *National Service Framework (NSF) for Children, Young People and Maternity Services* (Department of Health, 2004). The NSF was informed by scientific literature and recommendations from professionals and researchers in the field, which highlighted the importance of promoting normality and choice, and improving women's experiences of care.

To quote the NSF Standard 11 relating to maternity services:

'... women should be able to choose the most appropriate place and professional to attend during childbirth, based on her wishes and cultural preferences and any medical and obstetric needs that she or her baby may have.'

(Department of Health, 2005)

Summary

An analysis of the anthropological and historical perspectives has shown that women have been delivering in variations of the upright position for centuries, and left to their own accord would naturally assume the upright position for childbirth. In the 20th century, the medicalisation of childbirth played an important role in determining the type of care that women received in childbirth. Subsequently, this led to the 'medicalisation of birthing positions' as obstetricians took over the care of women in pregnancy, labour and childbirth. Government policies within the UK also dictated the kind of care that women would receive. In the 1970s a sudden rise in the rates of hospital delivery was shown to correlate with the rates of interventions imposed on women. Inevitably, the 'bed' became a central focus in the care of women in the clinical arena, which in turn led to a fall in the number of women who were encouraged to deliver in the upright position as more and more women were confined to the bed.

The influence of pressure groups led to a call for the humanisation of care delivery and a return to women-centred care, including giving women more choice and control and involving them in the decision-making process for their own care.

In the next chapter, the concept of choice, preferences and control will be discussed in relation to the theory that informed choice leads to knowledge empowerment, which in turn results in increased collaboration on decision-making between the woman and the midwife.

CHAPTER 4

Choice, preferences and control

In the spirit of democracy and openness, the *Good Birth Guide* was published as a supplement in a popular newspaper magazine (Foster, 2001). The guide included a detailed and comprehensive survey of all maternity units in the UK. Its main aim was to provide sufficient information to help women distinguish the type of care provided by each hospital – in other words, to help women make one of the most important decisions in their life. It was about giving women choice and control over their pregnancy and childbirth. Since the publication of the guide, women in the UK have been in a much better position to see the quality of care offered at their place of birth.

The guide also serves to heighten women's awareness of the variety of choices and options available to them. Unfortunately, what it does not do is explain how women go about making their choices and preferences known to the professionals who will be caring for them. Moreover, the quality and accuracy of the *Good Birth Guide* is only as good as the professionals who provide the information. However, the guide has recently been updated, and now provides more comprehensive data detailing where women can give birth and how they go about making their choices known to their GPs or midwives. It also provides updated maternity and birth statistics for each healthcare trust in the UK (Foster, 2005).

Much has been written on the woman's right to choose her place of birth (Campbell and MacFarlane, 1990; Tew, 1990; Dodwell and Armes, 2001), whether to have a caesarean or not (Hillan, 1996; Foster, 2001; Robinson, 2001) and whether to have epidural analgesia in labour or not (Bevis, 1999; Foster, 2001). However, a woman's right to choose her birthing position and take control of the decision-making process in childbirth has received minimal attention.

The *Good Birth Guide* (Foster, 2005) and the latest Department of Health NHS Maternity Statistics report for 2003-2004 (Government Statistical Service, 2005) may have provided useful statistics on current rates of caesarean section (23%), instrumental delivery (12%), induction (>20%), episiotomy (12%) and home birth (3%), but there was nothing on birthing positions. The question of whether women have the right to choose their birthing positions was not mentioned once in these reports; furthermore, only a few maternity units in the UK include this statistic in their annual report, suggesting that this option is low on their agenda (Coppen, 2002). In contrast, 'home-from-home' birth centres in the UK do provide statistics on the different types of birth positions adopted by women at the centres (Ackerman, 2002), intimating that these women are given a choice and that the use of different birthing positions is on their agenda.

While the *Good Birth Guide* does highlight one of the fundamental problems with childbirth care provision in the UK, namely that women lack information and awareness on their right to choose how, where and what kind of care they wish to receive, it cannot guarantee that women will get what they want.

Such knowledge will not be news to midwives or women. In 1993, the *Changing Childbirth* report, written by an Expert Maternity Group headed by Baroness Cumberlege (Department of Health, 1993), highlighted the importance of providing choice, control and continuity of care to women. The premise of this report, in emphasising to health professionals the importance of a woman-centred service, was that women should feel confident about receiving accurate and unbiased information and be assured of high-quality care.

In addition, two other points were made:

'The woman should feel secure in the knowledge that she can make her choice after full discussion of all the issues with the professionals involved in her care.'

'The woman should feel confident that the professionals would respect her right to choose her care on that basis.'
(Department of Health, 1993, pp. 5-6)

Unfortunately, the initial euphoria of midwives and their attempts to implement the proposals from this report were short lived, as it was quickly realised that such demands could not be met without adequate resources and an increase in staffing levels. Nonetheless, the spirit in which *Changing Childbirth* was written was genuine, and the report highlighted the importance of providing informed choice and giving women control over decision-making in pregnancy and childbirth – once the domain of obstetricians and midwives.

But how can midwives give women control and choice concerning birthing positions? Some organisations, such as the National Childbirth Trust (1995) and the Active Birth Centre (1995), have tried to address this question. Childbirth educators such as Schott (1994, 2003), Nolan (1998) and Robertson (1994) have also highlighted the importance of giving women more control in childbirth. The provision of free antenatal education by the NHS has not done enough to empower women and prepare them for childbirth (Hetherington, 1990; Lee and Shorten, 1999; Jansen and Blizzard, 1999; Murphy-Black, 1990; Enkin et al, 2000). Yet, Jamieson (1994), Robertson (2000) and Schott (2003) assert that it is through such education that midwives are in an ideal position to empower women.

Some antenatal classes do emphasise the importance of moving around during labour, the role of instinctive behaviour and selection of the best positions for labour (Williams and Booth, 1985; Nolan, 1998; Schott and Priest, 2002). Unfortunately, such classes are few and far between and most do not explain how women can be empowered to make their specific preferences known to their midwives, so that they can take control of the decision-making process.

Kelly et al (2001) emphasised the importance of women having control in childbirth, and identified 11 factors that provided high control:

○ Not being left alone at key times during labour
○ Having their birth wishes followed completely
○ A normal vaginal delivery
○ A home birth
○ An active position for delivery
○ Meeting midwives before delivery
○ Community midwifery antenatal care
○ Being delivered by a community midwife
○ Being cared for by the same midwife throughout labour
○ Having one midwife in labour or as few as possible
○ Ease of birth.

Six factors were identified as providing low control in childbirth:

○ Being delivered while lying flat on their back
○ Being left alone at key times during labour
○ Not having their birth wishes followed completely
○ An unplanned or emergency caesarean
○ Having five or more midwives providing care in labour
○ Having a fetal blood sample taken, internal fetal monitoring or pethidine following interventions in labour, a general anaesthetic or caesarean section.

Kelly et al (2001) highlighted three main factors as important: having a normal vaginal delivery, a home birth and an active birth position, e.g. being propped up, kneeling or sitting upright. Moreover, these three factors were significantly related to high levels of control in childbirth and demonstrated the importance of providing women with the kind of care that would allow them to take control in childbirth and give them more choices.

In relation to choice, a woman's right to choose her birthing position in childbirth should not be underestimated. There are numerous birthing positions a woman can choose from, and it can be argued that many women may find it difficult to make a decision based on the information currently provided in antenatal education. Attempts to educate and thus empower women through antenatal education classes have met with both success and failure. Booth (1996) highlighted the need to redesign, review and individualise classes to meet current challenges in practice.

Most NHS classes today concentrate on providing general information about labour, e.g. the use of coping strategies such as pain relief, controlled breathing patterns, comfort measures, the role of the partner in labour, caring for the newborn and coping with parenthood (Nolan and Hicks, 1997; Murphy Black, 1990; Jansen and Blizzard, 1999; Nolan, 1999; Enkin et al, 2000). In contrast, encouraging women to voice their preferences on choice of birthing options has not received equal attention in parent education. The exception is classes provided by the National Childbirth Trust (1995), the Active Birth Centre (1995) and proponents of natural childbirth such as Robertson (1994), Schott (1994) and Nolan (1998). This may be due to the significant difference in attitudes encouraged by these groups, observed by Enkin et al (2000). These authors suggested that community-sponsored childbirth education classes were structured to incorporate the interests of parents, whereas hospital-based classes were directed at explaining and justifying (rather than questioning) existing policies, offering alternatives, and helping parents to decide their own birth plans. Such inequality may be explained by the fact that the provision of antenatal education in the UK is variable and highly dependent on staffing levels, available resources and individual unit protocols and guidelines (Currel, 1990; Murphy-Black, 1990; Schott and Henley, 1996; Simkin and Enkin, 1989; Slade, 1996).

The problems of inconsistencies in the provision of information and fragmented care are therefore crucial issues for midwives. The need to help women make their preferences known is now greater than ever, as women are given more control over decision-making. How can women be assisted in making the right choice, tailored to their own personal needs and preferences?

Within antenatal education, the routine practice of encouraging women to write down their birth plan has been used as a catalyst to discuss women's preferences and choices in labour with the midwife. This practice is now widespread in the UK and Australia. However, completion of a birth plan does not guarantee that it will be followed. A population-based survey in Australia by Brown and Lumley (1998) found no significant association between the use of a birth plan and the degree of women's involvement in decision-making. In contrast, an investigation into the use and effects of birth plans and how women perceive them has shown that most women thought the process of completing the birth plan had been useful in allowing discussion of the available options beforehand (Whitford and Hillan, 1998). However, in this retrospective questionnaire survey of 143 primigravidae, half the women said that the birth plan did not make any difference to the amount of control they felt during labour.

According to Kitzinger (1999), birth plans are often rejected, ignored, trivialised or ridiculed by caregivers and may be appropriated by the medical system and used to obtain patient compliance. This is possibly due more to a breakdown in communication than to the midwife's ignorance of the mother's birth plan. Ley (1982a) pointed out that dissatisfaction with communication was the most consistent complaint put forward by patients. Many studies have commented on the problems of poor communication, often resulting in misunderstanding, complaints, anxiety or dissatisfaction (Ley, 1982b, 1988; MacLeod-Clark, 1985; Sherr, 1989; Murphy-Black, 1990; Kirkham, 1993; Nolan and Hicks, 1997).

Price (1998) pointed out that facilitating the writing of birth plans is an important part of midwifery care. However, the evidence supporting this practice is inconclusive and debatable, and shows that birth plans may not be the best way for women to identify their choice and communicate their preferences to midwives.

Is there a way to assure women that their needs and preferences will be met by caregivers? Will such assurance empower women to take control of their decision-making in childbirth? The research study presented in this book is an attempt to find an alternative method based on the hypothesis that the provision of focused information will enhance knowledge, reduce decisional conflict and empower women to take control of their decision-making in childbirth.

Defining choice, preferences and control

In order to understand the concept of choice, preferences and control in relation to birthing positions, it is important to define each component.

Choice: The *Oxford English Dictionary* (2000) defines choice as 'an act of choosing, the right or ability to choose, or a range from which to choose'.

Choosing between options is therefore a decisional act, and making a choice is a definition of decision-making. The hypothesis for this research study is that giving women a course of focused information on the benefits of the upright birthing position will put them in a better position to choose between the options for birthing positions, giving them control over their decision-making.

It is widely accepted by midwives (Coppen, 1997) that women have the right to choose whatever position they wish for the delivery of their baby. However, whether midwives encourage women to use their position of choice is unknown. Prince and Adams (1987) pointed out that midwives should be prepared to respond sympathetically to mothers who want to deliver in a squatting, standing or unconventional position.

Preference: The *Oxford English Dictionary* (2000) defines preference as 'a greater liking for one alternative over another or others, or a thing preferred'. Research on birthing positions has focused mainly on birth outcomes and satisfaction in labour. Identifying women's preference for one birth position over another has not been addressed, and therefore little is known about women's preferences from the various positions available to them. It may be widely assumed that women have the right to choose whatever position they wish; if this is the case, it would explain why this issue has received minimal attention.

Lewis (1990) pointed out that childbearing women's concerns and preferences have changed over time, and medical matters are not the only issues that concern women in childbirth. Lewis emphasised that the conflicting demands of the medical and the midwifery profession cannot be ignored. Obstetricians would view the childbirth process pathologically and only consider it 'normal' in retrospect, whereas midwives, who are generally optimists, would only interfere with childbirth if labour was not progressing well, and would view childbirth as a normal physiological event. Such conflicting demands and viewpoints may sometimes work against women during childbirth. As a result, women's preferences and concerns may sometimes be seen as unimportant and in conflict with the priorities of the medical and midwifery professions. If this is the case, what can be done to help women regain control of their childbirth?

Control: Control is defined by the *Oxford English Dictionary* (2000) as having the 'power to influence people's behaviour or the course of events'. In relation to giving women a choice of birthing positions and making their preferences known to the midwives caring for them, how helpful is the concept of control in helping women in their decision-making? Psychologists have proposed several theories in their attempts to conceptualise control. Two of the most quoted and long-standing concepts are locus of control (Rotter, 1966) and self-efficacy (Bandura, 1977).

Locus of control is defined as a person's belief about whether his or her behaviour can determine a certain outcome or not. Internal locus of control is the belief that one's own behaviour can control what happens, whereas external locus of control is the belief that the outcome is determined by chance or by powerful others (Weaver, 1998). Thus a woman who is informed about the choices of birthing position available to her would avail herself of this knowledge to her caregiver, and the outcome would be governed by the extent to which the woman's internal and external loci of control are accepted by her caregiver.

Wallston et al (1987), however, believed that locus of control says little about belief in what one should do. Also, it does not take into account issues such as the value of the outcome to the individual, the psychological issue at stake and the choices of alternative behaviour available in a given situation (Rotter, 1975).

Another concept of control, proposed by Bandura in the 1970s, is self-efficacy. Bandura (1977) suggests that behaviour is more likely to occur in the presence of three expectancies:

º When the woman believes that she has the ability to carry out the behaviour
º When she thinks she will bring about certain outcomes
º When she herself positively values these outcome expectancies.

In the context of giving a woman choice and preference over birthing positions, the woman must feel that she has the ability to carry them out by making her choices and preferences clear to her caregiver. The woman will also need to feel confident that making her preferences known to her caregiver will lead to certain outcomes, such as greater comfort, satisfaction, reduced pain, shorter labour and greater ability to push, and she must value these outcomes herself.

It is argued that existing methods of antenatal education do not help women to achieve self-efficacy to the fullest. Moreover, there is some debate as to whether it is more important to exert control or believe that one can exert control (Slade, 1996). Litt (1988) suggests that the latter may be more important in labour, and therefore the self-efficacy theory may be relevant. How can women be helped to apply the concept of self-efficacy in practice? I believes that self-efficacy can only occur if women are fully informed about the choices available to them and thus 'in control' of the decision-making. Foster (2001) pointed out the importance of making women feel in control of the birth process.

The concept of providing informed choice that will result in knowledge empowerment, reduced decisional conflict and greater control in decision-making will be discussed in the next section.

Informed choice as knowledge empowerment

Few professionals would argue about the benefits to be gained from informing women of the choices available to them so that they can make evidence-based decisions crucial to their individual needs. What is less clear is the best way to inform women about the choices of birthing position available to them. Dodwell and Armes (2001) pointed out that childbirth educators are only too aware that the majority of women have very little information on which to base their choice of maternity care and place of birth. This led to the launch of the website BirthChoiceUK.com (Dodwell and Armes, 2001) aimed at helping women to make informed choices.

Dodwell and Armes (2001) point out the obvious differences between antenatal education provided by the NHS and that provided by natural childbirth groups. For example, private classes such as those run by the National Childbirth Trust and the Active Birth antenatal education programmes are less structured, more flexible and include techniques for practising different positions in labour. By contrast, antenatal classes run by the NHS include information on what labour is like, pain relief, interventions and caesarean birth, but often exclude information on strategies for trying out different birthing positions in labour, in order to learn which position suits the woman best, which in turn will help her cope with labour. Thus a medical or prescriptive model of educating women would appear to exist within NHS classes, whereas a women-centred and flexible model of education is the norm in private classes. If this is the case, then the importance of having balanced and unbiased information provided by midwives cannot be accurately conveyed to women, since they are not fully informed about the choices available to them.

However, the fact that women are willing to pay to attend private antenatal classes suggests that NHS classes are not empowering women with the necessary knowledge for them to make an informed choice. Unfortunately, studies on the impact of antenatal education classes on women's knowledge and providing informed choice have been plagued by methodological limitations (Hillier and Slade, 1989). For example, Nunnally and Aguiar (1974) and Breese (1976) evaluated knowledge in the post-delivery period rather than at the end of the classes. Husband (1983) used a longitudinal design involving repeated measurements to assess the impact of antenatal classes on knowledge. Assessments were not made before and after the end of classes, but at first registration and before delivery, rendering the results spurious. Nevertheless, the knowledge level of attendees in this study increased by 10% over time compared with non-attendees, but the difference was small and the statistical measures used were not clear.

Hillier and Slade (1989) compared the impact of antenatal classes on knowledge, anxiety and confidence levels in hospital- and community-based groups of primiparous women. Sixty-seven women completed assessments of their knowledge, anxiety and confidence, before first attendance and after completion of the course. There was a highly significant increase in knowledge levels following the classes. Age and weeks of pregnancy at first attendance in the two groups were significantly different, with hospital attendees being significantly older and attending classes later. Initial knowledge levels were significantly associated with age, social class and educational level. Final knowledge levels were not significantly associated with these factors or with class size or number of classes attended. Knowledge and confidence levels showed substantial increases over the period of the classes. However, this was not a controlled trial as there was no control group of non-attendees. Therefore, it was not possible to establish a cause-and-effect relationship.

A Swedish study of women's perceptions of childbirth and childbirth education before and after education and birth by Hallgren et al (1995) found that women understood the content of education in different ways. Fear, as well as unreflected knowledge, appeared to block the acquisition of new knowledge. Lack of or inconsistent information contributed to a childbirth experience that was worse than expected, while increased knowledge about childbirth contributed to a good or better experience than expected. The authors concluded that consistency of information given before and during childbirth supports a sense of comprehensibility, manageability and meaningfulness. This reinforces the importance of providing adequate information to empower women with the necessary knowledge to make an informed choice.

Studies on the provision of informed choice in relation to birthing positions *per se* are limited. However, one important study was that of Oliver et al (1996) published by the NHS Centre for Reviews and Dissemination. A growing enthusiasm for some sort of intervention to help women make informed choices led to the development of this pilot project, which was carried out over a 6-month period in three London Hospitals. The authors assessed the value of 'informed choice' leaflets on positions in labour in assisting women in their decision-making. General questions, such as whether the leaflets were beneficial in helping women to increase their knowledge and who should be responsible for distributing the leaflets, were highlighted in the pilot study. More importantly, issues such as womens' involvement in decision-making during labour, effectiveness of the leaflet during labour and the positions of the women at the moment of giving birth were also highlighted. Thirty-seven midwives were involved in the distribution of the leaflets and 131 women were recruited to the study. Women were asked to answer a series of questions from a questionnaire survey following receipt of the information leaflet and during the postnatal period.

The results showed that although most women found the leaflets useful in keeping them informed about what was available, some pointed out that being informed did not necessarily lead to choice as they needed to be reminded about alternative upright positions when they were in labour. Failing that, they were more likely to adopt the conventional recumbent positions, thereby further reducing their choice and control in labour. Some women, who had been given an intravenous infusion and needed to stay in bed, commented on their lack of choice and option to move around and stay in the position of their choice. A worrying, but not surprising, finding in this study was that some women found out for the first time that they had a choice and that they could choose to deliver in upright positions. Some did not even realise that there were so many positions to choose from.

In their systematic review on positions for women in the second stage of labour, Gupta and Hofmeyr (2004) concluded that women should be encouraged to give birth in whatever position is comfortable for them. However, it is argued that unless women are first informed about the various options available to them and encouraged to attempt different birthing positions in labour, they may not know what is most comfortable for them.

Another woman in Oliver et al's study (1996) commented that the leaflet on informed choice was far too brief, and she would have liked more information on the props that one could use in labour. Some women thought that the pictures in the leaflet did not demonstrate all the possible positions that one could use, e.g. the squatting position. However, 23% of the women liked all the pictures, 41% said that the pictures showed them what to expect, and 13% said that the pictures did not show them what to expect. A participant who displayed her doubts and frustration about existing care provision made this poignant comment:

> 'How long will it take for hospitals to accept all this; we've had the vote long enough, it's about time we were allowed to choose how to have the baby.'

> (Oliver et al, 1996, p.14)

Despite the benefits of upright birthing positions highlighted in the leaflets, only a minority of women tried using the upright positions in labour. Of the 110 women finally entered into the study, only 56 responded. The different positions tried by these women during labour included lying on their back (54%), lying on their side (46%), sitting propped up (73%), standing up (45%), on all fours (18%), kneeling (20%) and squatting (11%); 9% used the birth pool and 5% used the bath during labour. A fifth (20%) of the women said that they did not get enough help with using birthing positions, although 48% did not have any difficulty getting into the positions they wanted. A third (30%) of women said they had wanted to try other positions but did not do so, either because they were too tired, because nobody suggested another position, or for some other reason.

Causes for concern were statements made by women who pointed out that they had no encouragement from their midwife and that there was a distinct lack of useful birthing apparatus, such as birth stools or birth balls, to help them maintain an upright position. An interesting finding in this study was the fact that monitoring of the fetal heart rate was a barrier to full choice of positions in labour. This suggests that midwives and obstetricians were not meeting the needs of women and that, once again, monitoring of women in labour superseded women's right to choose and to refuse procedures imposed on them.

The study also found a huge variation in the type of positions used in all three hospitals, ranging from a hospital where 19% of women were delivering on their backs, to another where 42% were doing so. Women who delivered on their backs were more likely to be primiparous and working class. Variations in the attitudes of staff, the delivery of care and the ease with which women were able to talk to the midwives about the information they had gained from the leaflets were also observed. The power struggle between women and their professional carers was also highlighted in this study, which showed that, despite the information given to the women, their increased knowledge did not help them in their decision-making. The study revealed that midwives did not necessarily reinforce the knowledge that the women had gained or encourage them to try different positions. This was something the women very much wanted, as they felt that during labour they forgot what they had read or learnt. The lack of reinforcement and encouragement by the midwives was highlighted by one participant, in the comment:

> 'The leaflet was very informative, but, as I explained, I was in a great deal of pain, and completely forgot about different positions. Perhaps the midwife or doctor should have suggested different positions.'
>
> (Oliver et al, 1996, p.18)

In contrast, midwives in this study responded to the use of the leaflets enthusiastically and were more optimistic about its influence in encouraging discussion. Eleven (79%) of the 14 midwives who responded to the questionnaire thought that the leaflet would help women to talk to midwives and doctors about their care, yet only 5% of women said the leaflet did so. However, 13% of the women felt that it helped them talk to their partner. Nine (64%) of the 14 midwives thought that the leaflet would help women make informed choices about positions in labour, yet only 24% of the women said that it helped them personally. No midwife thought that the information on birthing positions given in the leaflet affected the care or provision offered in their unit, although some thought that it might do so in the future. Some suggestions for changes were proposed, e.g. some midwives thought there was a need for greater distribution of the leaflets by other professionals such as health visitors; others thought that there should be better availability of props, and some suggested greater use of upright positions. Some midwives also intimated that positions in labour were discussed at antenatal classes, although Dodwell and Armes (2001) found that this was not the case.

Oliver et al (1996) have clearly shown that the use of leaflets on positions in labour to inform women and give them more choice and control over their labour was not as successful as had been hoped. This study also highlighted the resistance of some health professionals to the use of evidence-based health care, and that only a minority of women found the informed choice leaflets had helped them to labour in upright positions.

Underlying conflicts with the principle of professional autonomy were also apparent among midwives, who expressed concern that informed choice may create anxiety and professional and organisational barriers to allowing choice for women (Oliver et al, 1996). Yet Paterson-Brown, a female consultant obstetrician at Queen Charlotte's Hospital, London, believes that both doctors and midwives should be much more forthcoming with information to enable women to make an informed choice (Scott, 2001).

Discussing choice and options with women does not necessarily empower them with the knowledge, as the dissemination of knowledge by professionals can be fragmented and there is no agreement as to how much and what kind of information women need to possess (Jacoby, 1988; Kirkham, 1993; Oliver et al, 1996; Nolan, 1998). There also appears to be a socio-cultural bias in relation to how much information women are given (Cartwright, 1979; Kirkham, 1989; Schott and Henley, 1996). Moreover, some obstetricians and midwives are more forthcoming with their information, whereas others are more possessive of the knowledge.

The reluctance of medical and midwifery staff to disseminate information may be due to the existence of a hidden agenda – the belief that 'knowledge is power' and the release of such knowledge can lead to apparent powerlessness.

Jordan (1993), in her extensive study on authoritative knowledge regarding birth, found that certain individuals appear to be authoritative because of the knowledge they possess. Jordan found that the one with the greater knowledge would take precedent over those with less knowledge. Thus it may be assumed that the midwife or obstetrician, by virtue of their training and education, would possess greater knowledge about midwifery or obstetrics than the mother in labour. Such authoritative knowledge is accepted as legitimate, is socially sanctioned and serves as grounds for action (Sargent and Bascope, 1996). This highlights the power of authoritative knowledge and provides some explanation for the continuing struggle between professionals and clients in relation to choice, control and decision-making in labour. The respect accorded to authoritative knowledge legitimises the control of action (Sargent and Bascope, 1996) and implies ownership of some status, quality or claim that compels trust and obedience (Starr, 1982). It is this authority and status of authoritative knowledge conferred on professionals that allows them to make judgments and decisions about what is best for women, and the role of women is to listen and comply (Sargent and Bascope, 1996).

Such authoritative knowledge does not seem to sit comfortably in today's climate of women-centred care. The concept of authoritative knowledge has been researched in the anthropological field (Young, 1982; Clifford and Marcus, 1986; Marcus and Fischer, 1986; Kaufert and O'Neil, 1993; Rapp, 1993), which looked at the status of biomedicine as a realm of knowledge that is valid and authoritative but separate from other socio-cultural domains. However, some authors (e.g. Rhodes,1990; Lindenbaum and Lock, 1993) have argued that the legitimisation of such knowledge is in itself a cultural process.

Jordan's (1993) study of authoritative knowledge in childbirth also demonstrated the priorities that physicians assigned to technology and birth procedures and less so to the competing kind of knowledge held by women. Authoritative knowledge was also shown to be produced through social interactions and hierarchically distributed. Because of this process of interaction, technological knowledge becomes the knowledge that 'counts' and on which decisions are based (Sargent and Bascope, 1996). While Jordan (1997) argued that authoritative knowledge is possessed by those who control and dominate it, Sargent and Bascope (1996) proposed that authoritative knowledge is contingent on shared experience, social position and the birth setting. In their anthropological study of women in labour, they found that the authoritative knowledge of the midwife was less important or visible in a multigravid woman, compared with a woman who was experiencing her first birth. The woman experiencing her first labour was considered inexperienced and therefore unable to cope with labour herself – this legitimised the position of the midwife in possessing greater knowledge and therefore controlling how the labour should progress.

Sargent and Bascope (1996) also showed that in a collaborative and low technology birthing system, the midwife and woman in labour often share the knowledge and negotiate the terms of the woman's care. In a high technology birthing system, however, the reverse is true – some women expect a medicalised childbirth and respect the professionals' knowledge of their care, thereby assuming a weaker position of power and control over their body and the decision-making process (Jordan and Irwin, 1989; Sargent and Bascope, 1996).

The studies on authoritative knowledge discussed thus far do not address what will happen when informed choice is afforded to the women. Whether a shift in power and thus of authoritative knowledge, or a collaborative state of decision-making, as found in Sargent and Bascope's study, will occur remains to be seen. It is interesting that a recent qualitative study of how midwives facilitate informed choice and women make informed choices in pregnancy highlighted the issues of power that permeated the data, where the dominant group controls what may or may not be discussed and therefore what decisions may be made (Levy, 1999a,b,c). Hence a shift in the balance of power, and thus knowledge, is long overdue. Such radical changes and shift in the balance of power reinforce the need for greater collaboration between midwives and women in relation to decision-making.

Professionals need only turn to the numerous reports and calls for reform published by successive governments to realise the need for change. Two such reports are *Changing Childbirth* (Department of Health, 1993), which called for a return to giving women choice, control and continuity, and *The New NHS: Modern, dependable* (Department of Health, 1997), which called for a rethink on the way that health professionals are providing care. The creation of a National Service Framework aimed at progressive and effective delivery of care (Maternity Care Working Party, 2000) and the Audit Commission's *First Class Delivery* (1997) emphasised the central position that women should play in pregnancy and childbirth. Collectively, all these reports are asking for the same fundamental change, namely a shift in the balance of power towards women-centred care and away from professional-centred control. They are calling for a partnership in healthcare delivery.

In this climate of change, the time is right to consider a radical change – an alternative and innovative method of informing women about the choices of birthing position available to them. The change would authorise and empower women with the knowledge they need to make an evidence-based decision regarding their choice of positions in labour.

As discussed earlier, the degree to which women are expected to make an informed choice, based on the current fragmented and variable provision of information, has been criticised. An ethnographic study designed to examine the effects of informed choice found that informed choice, as it is currently received, may not lead to any changes in childbirth experience for women, owing to the cultural needs of women in society, which have not been met (Machin and Scamell, 1998).

The value of informed choice has also been questioned in a report that highlighted the importance of building up a trusting relationship over time between the midwife and the parent if informed choice is to be successful (Anderson and Rosser, 1998). Moreover, informed choice for black women and women from ethnic minorities has not been addressed sufficiently as most initiatives in research studies are designed for white women who can speak and read English. This is a common feature in most Western research today (Turner et al, 1996).

In contrast, Churchill and Benbow (2000) investigated informed choice within maternity services in Powys, Wales, in relation to the caregiver and location of care. They found high levels of satisfaction with the amount of information on antenatal and birth care received by women in the study. Midwives were identified as playing an essential role in informing women in all antenatal and birth settings. Moreover, midwives in midwife-led antenatal clinics and midwife/GP maternity units were more successful in imparting information and enabling women to have a sense of participation in the decision-making process. This study showed that organisational or experiential factors have a greater impact on women's perceptions of having an active role in the decision-making process than the healthcare personnel involved.

In another study, Newburn (2000) focused on the complex issues involved in providing informed choice, and found that the most significant factor determining the success of informed choice was time. The amount of time that midwives have available to listen to women and advise them is limited (Newburn, 2000). Similarly, Price (1998) described the difficulty of advocating choice to women in a situation where it is unlikely to be fulfilled owing to time constraints. However, one could argue that a midwife who is sensitive to the needs of individual women would surely not deprive them of the appropriate information and advice, regardless of any time constraints.

A series of studies by Levy (1999a,b,c) looked at the processes involved when midwives engaged in facilitating the making of informed choices by women in the UK. A grounded theory approach was used to draw on the interactions that occur between the midwives and the women. The study found that a core category identified as 'protective steering' occurred, where midwives were concerned with protecting women in their care, gate keeping and raising awareness. Levy (1999b,d) also found that, at the same time, a woman would attempt to make choices that would preserve the balance of her life and that of her family. The core category identified in this was 'maintaining equilibrium'. In this latter study, Levy noted that women judged the trustworthiness of the information given by the midwife before making their choices. It is therefore important for midwives to build up a trusting relationship with the women to allow them to reach their own decisions about how best to 'maintain their equilibrium'. Studies by Levy (1999a,b,c,d) reinforce the need for health professionals to empower and assist women in their decision-making, thereby facilitating informed choices.

Informed choice in maternity services is also dependent on the confidence of the women to exercise choice and assert their wishes (Churchill and Benbow, 2000). In their quantitative survey of 215 women, Churchill and Benbow identified midwives as the primary source of information. Most women in the study perceived that they had high levels of informed decision-making. The majority of women (77%) said that they were encouraged to make informed decisions about their care during labour, and 83% felt that they had taken an active part in decision-making about the birth of their baby. However, this survey did not identify the information given to the women, and it may be that their perception of feeling informed was related to their high satisfaction with the childbirth experience.

Machin and Scamell (1998), in a scathing report about the way informed choice is provided through antenatal education, revealed that it is at best superficial and at worst an illogical method. The women in this study felt that the information given to them in their antenatal classes did not reflect the reality of what happens in the labour ward. All their choices were either ignored or rendered irrelevant as they were subsumed by medical procedures. All the women felt vulnerable and handed over responsibility to the professionals. This study suggests that women lose their autonomy, control and decision-making power in labour, and a change in the way that antenatal education is provided is needed as a matter of urgency to address this.

Robertson (2000) commented that the concept of informed choice in maternity care is a mirage, and that parents are often encouraged to make decisions before they are fully informed. She highlighted the need for childbirth educators to provide parents with the necessary information so that they can make an informed choice about their care, even though that choice may be contrary to midwives' preferences.

Summary

The concept of choice, the need to give women control over their bodies and identification of women's preferences are complex issues that cannot be resolved simply by providing antenatal education. Variation in the delivery of information and dissemination of knowledge from professional carers to women are central to the problems that prevent women from choosing their birthing positions and making their preferences known. The influence of authoritative knowledge on women's ability to make decisions highlights the control and power that professionals have over women in relation to knowledge acquisition.

Informed choice is of value in providing knowledge empowerment, which is seen as an important method of giving women greater choice, control and autonomy. However, health professionals also need to recognise that there are limitations to providing informed choice, especially when the balance of power (and of knowledge) remains in the hands of health professionals and not the women in their care.

Midwives may need to seek alternative ways of disseminating information and increasing women's control and choice in childbirth. In clinical practice today, women need to be more empowered to make their choices regarding birthing positions known and their voices heard, especially during delivery, one of the most vulnerable stages of their pregnancy. It is proposed that a collaborative approach to decision-making – a form of shared decision-making – may be an effective alternative.

The next chapter discusses the concept of collaborative decision-making and highlights Roger's innovation-decision model as a theoretical framework in support of the research process (Rogers, 1995). The development of ADAPT (a decision anaylsis preference triage), an instrument or tool to help women make decisions about their choice of birthing positions, will then be discusssed. I believe that women want to know all about the use of different birthing positions, and want to be encouraged by their midwives and carers. Women also want to be in control and be empowered to make their own decisions about their choice of birthing position. I hope they will find ADAPT useful in helping them to meet their individual needs concerning their choice of birthing positions.

CHAPTER 5

Collaborative decision-making

The importance of giving women choice, identifying their preferences and giving them control over their childbirth was discussed at length in chapter 4, and weaknesses in the way that information is disseminated to women in pregnancy were highlighted. The chapter concluded that an alternative method of disseminating evidence-based information to women was needed. A collaborative decision-making approach via the provision of focused information was proposed.

In this chapter I will discuss Rogers' (1995) innovation-diffusion theory – an aspect of behavioural decision theory – in relation to choice of birthing positions, as a possible aid to eliciting women's values of a given option. A new decision aid applicable to midwifery practice to help women with the decision process concerning choice of birthing positions will be introduced. The development of a decision-analysis preference triage (ADAPT), as a new decision aid (instrument) to guide women's decisions regarding birth positions, will be examined in relation to how it can be applied to maximise and identify women's choices, thereby promoting a holistic approach to collaborative decision-making.

Women are still delivering in recumbent positions today because they are not given sufficient information about the available alternatives. It is proposed that these alternatives may be the better choice/option for the individual woman concerned. Giving women more choice and more information is an important issue in midwifery care today. However, before women can make a choice, they need to know what the alternatives are. Once they have this knowledge, women are empowered to make their decisions known to their midwives, which in turn fosters collaborative decision-making between the midwife and the woman.

> *'It could be argued that the single most important skill needed*
> *by a new parent is the ability to make decisions.'*
>
> (Robertson, 1994, p.63)

Innovation-diffusion theory of decision-making

Pregnant women have to make crucial decisions about their health and welfare during pregnancy, labour and the postnatal period. They face uncertainties, decision options and a proliferation of information during pregnancy.

Roger's (1995) innovation-diffusion theory of decision-making is based on the important concepts of uncertainty and information. Rogers theorised that uncertainty in a given situation is due to a weakness in the diffusion of ideas, and identified five stages in the innovation-decision process through which an individual must pass before moving to the next stage. He defines uncertainty as the degree to which a number of alternatives are perceived with respect to the occurrence of an event, and the relative probabilities of those alternatives.

Within the area of midwifery that we are discussing, 'delivery position' is the event that women will be considering as options and alternatives that they may choose from. I concur with Rogers (1995) that uncertainty may be a good thing as it motivates an individual to seek information, it implies a lack of predictability of the structure of information, and information giving is a process that affects uncertainty in a situation where a choice exists among a set of alternatives. Given that women's uncertainty about their choice of birthing positions was related to a lack of information about birth positions, Rogers and Kincaid (1981) defined the process of uncertainty as a difference in 'matter-energy' (which I prefer to call the 'uncertainty gap'). They argued, therefore, that the way to address the problems arising from the difference in 'matter-energy', which exist in giving information, is to provide focused information to women to assist them in their choice and decision-making.

An innovation is any new action, idea or product (*Oxford English Dictionary,* 2000) or an idea that is perceived as new, although not necessarily in terms of chronology (Rogers, 1983). Diffusion, according to Rogers, is the process by which an innovation is communicated through certain channels over time among the members of a social system. It is a special type of communication in which the messages are concerned with new ideas. According to Hanson (1998a, 1998b), innovation-diffusion theory can also be applied to the study of new ideas and their dissemination among providers of care; I would add that recipients of health care may also benefit from the study of new ideas. Diffusion is a kind of social change, defined as the process by which alteration occurs in the structure and function of a social system. Rogers believed that when new ideas are invented, diffused and adopted or rejected, it leads to certain consequences and a degree of social change.

In this research, I propose to use a strategy – 'focused information' (*the innovation*) – to encourage women to be more aware of the research evidence and choices available to them with respect to alternative positions in labour. I believe that women need to be fully informed before they can make a sound decision and choice (*the diffusion*) appropriate to their individual needs. The decision or choice that the woman makes, i.e. to adopt the upright position or not, is in a sense a 'social change' for her, and for the midwives who care for her, because it may involve a move away from the norm and established ideas.

The rationale behind the innovation (focused information) is that women are often uncertain about the choices available to them, and need to be given the information in order to reduce the uncertainty. Innovations often take many years to plan and many more years in testing before they are adopted (Rogers, 1995). Rogers' concept of the innovation-diffusion theory is thus to speed up this lengthy process so that the innovation is accepted more readily and more quickly in order to benefit the people who would use it.

The five stages in Rogers' innovation-decision process, through which an individual passes, are as follows:

° First knowledge of an innovation
° Forming an attitude towards the innovation
° Decision to adopt or reject the innovation
° Implementation of the new idea
° Confirmation of this decision.

This process consists of a series of actions and choices over time, through which an individual evaluates a new idea and decides whether to incorporate the new idea to meet his/her individual needs. This involves dealing with the uncertainty that is inherent in deciding about a new alternative – in this case, the woman's choice to use an alternative position for delivery, based on the evidence shown. The woman will either adopt or reject the new information. If she adopts the information, it is hoped that her choice of birthing position will be implemented in collaboration with the midwife who cares for her. Depending on individual circumstances, the midwife will confirm whether or not the mother's decision, and therefore her preference, can be accommodated; however, if the midwife gives out conflicting messages about the value of using upright positions, this may lead to rejection of the innovation by the woman.

These five stages may be represented by a model of the innovation-decision process adapted from Rogers' (1995) model:

1. **Knowledge** occurs when an individual is exposed to an innovation's existence and gains some understanding of the evidence for and against the innovation (use of the upright position). At this stage, the knowledge or skills for effective adoption of the innovation are acquired. The exposure in this case is the provision of focused information on the use of upright birthing positions to the women.

2. **Persuasion** occurs when an individual forms a favourable or unfavourable attitude towards the innovation. The researcher's role is crucial during this stage as the women seek to evaluate the usefulness of the innovation in reducing uncertainty by asking for more information before making a decision. The researcher has the greatest opportunity to persuade the women to take the best course of action according to evidence-based practice at this stage of the decision process.

3. **Decision** occurs when an individual engages in activities that lead to a choice to adopt or reject the innovation. At this stage, the woman makes a decision without the influence of the researcher. The 'activities' engaged in by the women could take the form of completion of a questionnaire, or the decision analysis instrument ADAPT. In addition, women may also discuss their options with the midwife who will care for them in labour before accepting or rejecting the innovation. (The use of ADAPT will be discussed in the next section.)

4. **Implementation** occurs when an individual puts an innovation into use. This will occur during labour when the woman makes her decision explicit to her midwife. Women may or may not seek additional information about the use of the upright position from the midwife before implementation. Collaborative decision-making is required for successful implementation to take place.

5. **Confirmation** occurs when an individual seeks reinforcement of an innovation decision already made, or reverses a previous decision to adopt or reject the innovation if exposed to conflicting messages about the innovation. By this stage a firm decision would be made by the woman in collaboration with the midwife. Recognition of the benefits of using the innovation (upright position) and promotion of the innovation to other women usually occurs at this stage, once the innovation is adopted (McGuire, 1989).

According to Rogers (1995), it was assumed that persuasion would lead to a subsequent change in overt behaviour, i.e. adoption or rejection of the idea; in many cases, however, there seemed to be a discrepancy between attitudes and actions. For example, in a survey of Third World nations on family planning, Rogers (1973) found that although many parents of childbearing age had a favourable attitude towards the use of contraceptives, only 15–20% of individuals actually adopted the idea. The same can be said to have occurred with midwives in the use of birthing positions: although many midwives had a favourable attitude towards the use of non-lithotomy positions, in practice the number of midwives who actually adopted upright positions was lower than expected (Hanson, 1998a, 1998b).

Rogers (1973) referred to the discrepancy between attitude and change in adoption rate as the knowledge-attitude-practice (KAP) gap. Poor communication channels were identified as one reason for the KAP gap in the innovation-decision process: individuals were more likely to adopt the innovation if the information and communication channels were more open and available to the individual. It is this that prompted the researcher to attempt to narrow the gap by intoducing focused information as an innovation to midwifery practice, thereby providing women with informed choice.

The innovation-decision process is an information-seeking and information-processing activity in which women are motivated to reduce uncertainty about the advantages and disadvantages of the innovation (Rogers, 1995). Prior experience could influence a woman's decision to accept or reject the innovation, e.g. a woman who has had a previous traumatic delivery in the upright position is unlikely to adopt this position again. The change agent should meet the needs and address the problems of the woman before the persuasion stage takes place. For example, if a woman would like to deliver in the upright position but does not know how to go about it, then the change agent could reassure the woman by identifying all the different upright positions that the woman may be able to adopt during labour. Innovativeness is dependent on the change agent's ability to convince the woman of the value of using upright positions in labour. Norms present in midwifery practice can also influence the adoption or rejection of the innovation. For example, if the midwife prefers the recumbent position to the upright position, the woman could be influenced by this and thus be more likely to reject the innovation.

Certain behaviours are associated with each of the five stages in the innovation-decision process. As the change agent, the researcher would seek to create an 'awareness knowledge' about the innovation, i.e. the focused information on birthing positions. More importantly, the change agent will be considered to have done a better job of ensuring adoption of the innovation by teaching and motivating women on the 'how to knowledge', i.e. how upright positions can best be used in labour.

Empirical evidence of the validity of each stage in the innovation-decision process can be found in the Iowa study of farmers (Beal and Rogers, 1960), where respondents moved from awareness knowledge to a decision to adopt the innovation. This study also showed that respondents may be slow to adopt the innovation and the decision to adopt can occur over time; in the context of the present study, this would mean that although some women may decide not to adopt the upright position before labour, the decision to use it may be made during labour.

Figure 5.1 illustrates the five stages in the innovation-decision process.

A decision analysis preference triage (ADAPT)

There is very little published literature on how midwives and women decide which delivery position suits women best. Thus several important questions remain unanswered:

° What do women want in labour?
° Do women know all the available options when it comes to the different types of delivery positions?
° Do midwives know what is best for women in labour?

Most of the studies investigating decision aids have looked at how patients make decisions in the face of moral, ethical or serious dilemmas (e.g. Clancy et al, 1988; Haidet et al, 1998; Lilford et al, 1998; O'Connor et al, 1999). Decision aids help women to make specific and deliberative choices by providing information on the range of options available, and the benefits of each option (O'Connor et al, 2001, 2003). Decision aids can include other information about a given option, such as evidence of recent experience by other women, and research-based evidence on the benefits of its use. Such aids range from a simple information leaflet, to videos, tapes, media and computer programs and printed material (NHS Centre for Reviews and Dissemination, 2001; O'Connor et al, 2003).

The effectiveness of decision aids has been assessed in three main reviews (Molenaar et al, 2000; Estabrooks et al, 2001; O'Connor et al, 2003), none of which relates to midwifery issues. To date, no studies have been published on the use of a decision aid and focused education to help women identify their preferences regarding delivery position. A recent Cochrane Review (Horey et al, 2004) examining the effectiveness of methods used to inform women about caesarean section did include educating women about the options available as an important issue. Thus began my quest to develop a research strategy to inform women of the benefits of the upright posture for labour and

Figure 5.1: Model of the stages in the innovation-decision process (adapted from Rogers, 1995).

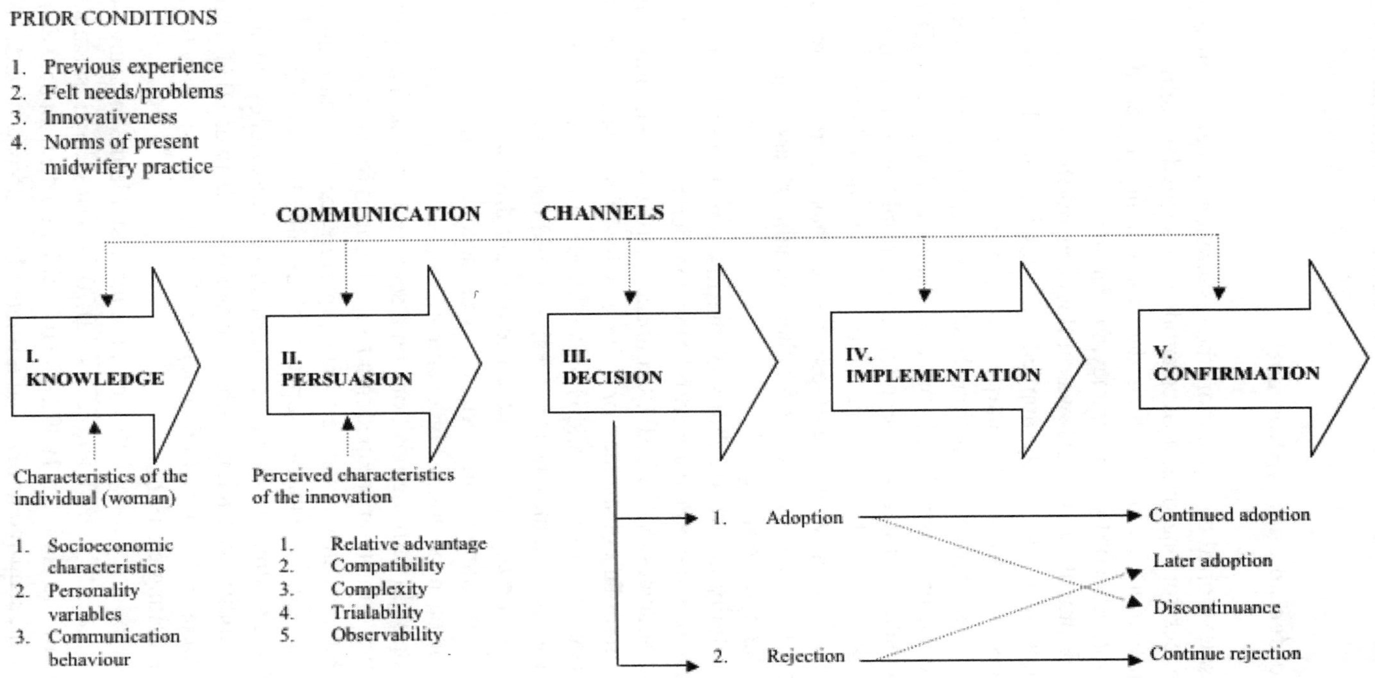

PRIOR CONDITIONS

1. Previous experience
2. Felt needs/problems
3. Innovativeness
4. Norms of present midwifery practice

COMMUNICATION   CHANNELS

I. KNOWLEDGE

Characteristics of the individual (woman)

1. Socioeconomic characteristics
2. Personality variables
3. Communication behaviour

II. PERSUASION

Perceived characteristics of the innovation

1. Relative advantage
2. Compatibility
3. Complexity
4. Trialability
5. Observability

III. DECISION

1. Adoption
2. Rejection

IV. IMPLEMENTATION

V. CONFIRMATION

Continued adoption

Later adoption

Discontinuance

Continue rejection

The *innovation-decision process* is the process through which an individual passes from first knowledge of an innovation, to forming an attitude towards the innovation, to a decision to adopt or reject, to implementation of the new idea, and confirmation of this decision.

delivery so that they can be empowered to collaborate on their decision and personal preference with the midwife who is caring for them during childbirth.

ADAPT as a decision aid (instrument)

ADAPT was developed by the author (the researcher) to help women highlight their preferences for one option over another. A secondary aim was to assist midwives in helping women in their decision-making, especially during the most vulnerable time of their pregnancy, i.e. labour.

The development of ADAPT was influenced by the need for a decision instrument that could be easily applied by midwives in clinical practice to enhance decision-making. The purpose of the instrument was to identify preferences for a particular position, based on eight possible positions that women could use to deliver their baby. The objective of applying ADAPT is to help women make their decisions explicit and to think through their choices by rating their top three preferences. In so doing, it was hoped that the women in the experimental group would be empowered to make their choices known to the midwife who would be caring for them in labour, based on the evidence presented to them in the study.

Internal validity and repeatability of the instrument were measured using Cronbach's alpha and the Pearson correlation coefficient via Statistical Package for the Social Sciences (SPSS 10.0). Cronbach's alpha is a reliability index that estimates the internal consistency or homogeneity of a measure composed of several items or subparts (Polit and Hungler, 1999). It is therefore an indication of how well a set of variables measures a single unidimensional latent construct. However, the nature of enquiry on the use of eight different birthing positions meant that a multidimensional structure was needed to determine women's preferences for each position. For example, women were asked to rate their preferences for eight birthing positions on a scale of 0–100%. The preferences for each position were then grouped into five categories for analysis: very weak, weak, no preference, strong and very strong preference. This multidimensional structure means that Cronbach's alpha will usually be low (UCLA, 2001). Using Cronbach's alpha to estimate the internal consistency of a measure produces a reliability coefficient with a normal range between 0.00 and +1.00, with higher values reflecting a higher degree of internal consistency (Cronbach, 1990; Polit and Hungler, 1999).

The higher the reliability coefficient, the more stable the measure; for most purposes a reliability coefficient above 0.70 is considered satisfactory or acceptable (Polit and Hungler, 1999). The reliability coefficient between the use of the recumbent, semi-recumbent and left lateral positions was 0.55. However, when analysed in relation to recumbent and semi-recumbent position,

Cronbach's alpha was higher at 0.60. When the upright positions, such as the kneeling, standing, squatting, semi-squatting and all-fours positions, were grouped together, Cronbach's alpha measured 0.82, demonstrating a significantly high degree of correlation. This means that the measurement of internal consistency was appropriate for the use of upright positions, but less so for recumbent positions. However, in some cases a higher coefficient may be required, or a lower one may be considered acceptable (Cronbach, 1990). It is argued that, on the whole, the internal reliability coefficient is acceptable because the uniqueness of the ADAPT instrument serves to measure a woman's preference for one type of position over another over a short period of time.

The differences in internal consistency between recumbent and upright positions reflect the distinct differences between these two groups. It may be that women's choices for recumbent positions were more tentative and hence did not reliably reflect their true preference. In contrast, for some women, deciding between the recumbent, semi-recumbent or left lateral positions was more of a certainty.

The ADAPT questionnaire (*Appendix 1*) is in two parts. Part 1 consists of five questions that women could respond to by ticking the box that most reflected their answers. In the first question, women were asked to rate their knowledge of birth positions following the intervention. The second question required the women to rate their preferences for one position over another on a scale of 0–100%. Women were also asked the reasons for their choice of birthing positions, based on five possible reasons. This question included an additional 'box', which allowed any other reason to be identified by the women. They were also asked to state how important it was for them to be able to use their choice of position for delivery. The purpose of this was to assess to what extent identifying their preference for a particular position was important to the women, as this would have implications for practice.

Part 2 of the questionnaire comprised two questions. The first was a rating scale to identify the women's knowledge of pain relief. In the second question, women were asked to rate their views of six different choices of pain relief. This was written into the questionnaire for the purpose of the randomised controlled trial. Participants were divided into control and experimental groups. The control group was given general information on pain relief, and the experimental group was given information focusing on positions in labour based on current evidence.

The use of ADAPT fits well into the five stages of the innovation-decision process, through which an individual must pass, as described by Rogers (1995). First, women in the experimental group would experience knowledge of the innovation, i.e. the focused information on birthing positions. Second, they would form an attitude or preference towards the innovation. This stage may occur during the course of the session at any point from listening to the research evidence on the use of upright positions to watching a 12-minute video of a woman delivering in the upright standing position. Some women may not have formed an attitude or preference towards the use of upright positions until the end of the session when they were given an opportunity to ask questions or express any concerns they may have had about birthing positions. Women's preferences for or against the use of an upright position may be swayed one way or another at the second stage. In the third stage, women were shown how to use the ADAPT instrument to help them in their decision-making, for it is at this stage that the woman would choose to adopt or reject the use of upright positions.

The principle behind the development of ADAPT was to assist women in identifying their preferences for each position. Following the weighing up of all eight possible positions that a woman could adopt or reject, all respondents were asked to note their top three preferences for labour. However, whether or not women would implement their decision (Rogers' fourth stage) or confirm that they were able to use their position of choice (Rogers' fifth stage) could not be identified until the end of labour when the participants completed a follow-up questionnaire (*Appendix 4*). The value of ADAPT as a valid instrument for decision-making will be discussed in the results section.

ADAPT is easy to complete and can be used by any woman as an aid to decision-making. It helps women express their wishes and plans during labour explicitly. ADAPT is especially beneficial for women who have definite ideas or wishes for a particular type of birthing position. The questionnaire identifies at a glance a woman's highest preference for a particular position, and would therefore be a useful instrument or tool for the midwife to use and apply in practice. ADAPT also makes it clear to the midwife what women want and what their preferences are before they go into labour. Of course, the nature of ADAPT is such that any woman may change her preference when she is in labour and may adjust her wishes accordingly in collaboration with her midwife. There is no rigidity in this plan – it is a decision aid, which, as the acronym implies, is also adaptable and flexible and can be adjusted to meet the needs of every woman. ADAPT can therefore play a pivotal role in labour.

ADAPT can also be used to include decision preference for other aspects of care, such as choice of pain relief. Some women, for example, may find it difficult to decide whether to have epidural analgesia or not. Others prefer to wait and see if they can cope with labour pains before making a decision – a view that I thoroughly support. It is with some regret that epidural analgesia has become a form of pain relief that is adopted all too easily by professionals and women in labour. No-one knows the long-term effect of epidural analgesia in terms of whether women are worse off in later life for not experiencing the pains of labour. Moreover, there is evidence to show that women who opt for epidural analgesia experience longer labour, reduced uterine function, fetal malposition, increased risk of fever, increased use of oxytocin and are more likely to end up with an instrumental delivery (Goodfellow et al, 1983; Bates and Helm, 1985; Bates et al, 1985; Newton et al, 1995; Howell, 2000, 2004; Downe et al, 2004; Liu and Sia, 2004). This raises the question of whether every woman should be encouraged to complete ADAPT before deciding on epidural analgesia as the only form of pain relief in labour. This might encourage women to think more about the pros and cons, while also giving practitioners the opportunity to discuss possible side-effects and complications.

I am not trying to discourage the use of epidural anagesia *per se,* as it has been shown to be an effective form of pain relief (Howell, 2000, 2004; Liu and Sia, 2004), but I am strongly suggesting that midwives should encourage women to try alternative methods of pain relief, such as relaxation in water, massage or adopting an upright posture, before advocating the use of epidural analgesia. This form of analgesia should only be used as a last resort after other less invasive methods have been tried. I would add that 'mobile epidural' is preferable to the non-mobile variety, since mobile epidural has been shown to increase the chance of a normal birth (COMET, 2001). However, the chance of a normal birth with mobile epidural is still not as good as that in women who are not using epidural analgesia.

Systematic literature review

A systematic review of the literature was undertaken to identify the extent to which the evidence for and against the use of recumbent and upright positions during labour influences women's preferences and choice of birthing positions. Details of the systematic literature review will be published elsewhere in journals, but a summary will be included here. A total of 105 papers were reviewed. Gaps in the literature on birth positions, including the midwife's role in facilitating greater choice and decision-making with women regarding the use of different positions in labour and childbirth, were identified.

Discussion

The aim of the systematic review was to identify studies on: the pros and cons of recumbent and upright positions for childbirth; women's and professionals' views and preferences in relation to birthing positions; and the rationale for using recumbent or upright positions, including choice and the decision-making process. Historical and anthropological studies were included in the review to determine whether women had any preference for a particular birth position and whether any particular position could be identified as 'the natural position' to inform present practice. The review set out to identify gaps in the literature regarding the use of different positions for childbirth, and to highlight areas in need of further research.

Several studies in the review highlighted the need for midwives to encourage women to maintain the upright posture. Yet the conventional recumbent, semi-recumbent and lithotomy postures are still in use today. This suggests that women are not receiving sufficient encouragement regarding the positive aspects of using the upright posture during labour. The review also found very few studies on how mothers could be encouraged to deliver in the upright posture. Midwives who are reluctant to deliver in the upright posture are less likely to encourage women to deliver in this position. Walsh (2000) reinforced this point, citing it as one of the reasons for the continuing trend to deliver in the recumbent position in UK hospitals today.

Historical and anthropological accounts have shown that women continued delivering their babies in upright positions until the mid-19th century. Many women in both primitive and civilised cultures considered the use of upright postures, such as the kneeling, squatting and standing positions, natural and instinctive. Several studies reported that it was the influence of Western culture, together with the advent of obstetric intervention, that superseded an intuitive and natural birthing process which included the instinct to move to an upright posture to deliver a baby (Englemann, 1882; Rigby, 1857; Jarcho, 1934; Naroll et al, 1961; Wolf, 1988; Kleine-Tebbe et al, 1996).

There was a dearth of studies on decision-making regarding women's choice of birthing positions. The studies that were reported were descriptive and anecdotal. The majority of the descriptive studies and non-randomised studies revealed that many women wished to adopt the upright positions for subsequent pregnancies. This suggests that they had experienced positive aspects of using the upright positions in previous births, despite evidence showing increased blood loss and labial tears with these postures. However, no studies on women's awareness of the benefits of using an upright posture for childbirth were found, indicating a gap in the literature and the need to conduct studies to examine women's views and knowledge regarding the benefits of upright birthing positions. Indeed, Gardosi et al (1989b) pointed out that enthusiastic midwives were the ones who encouraged women to use an upright posture, and that women are not aware that there are several alternative positions that they can adopt to deliver their baby in the second stage of labour. Consequently, women become accustomed to expect to deliver in a recumbent position in the UK today.

The need to educate women and inform them about the benefits of using the upright posture was identified in several studies (McKay, 1980, 1984; Gupta and Lilford, 1987; Gupta et al, 1989a, 1989b; Waldenstrom and Gottval, 1991; De Jong et al, 1997; Coppen, 1999, 2002; De Jonge and Lagro-Janssen, 2004).

De Jonge and Lagro-Janssen (2004), for example, pointed out that midwives were the most important factor influencing the choice of birthing positions, yet McKay (1984) noted that, for some midwives, a move away from the traditional practice of delivering women in the supine, dorsal or recumbent positions could be threatening. Investment in time, patience and education may be required for positive change to occur in practice.

The review also found that attitude change towards the use of upright birthing postures needed to occur before midwives would adopt them. A survey of midwives' practice in Singapore (Coppen, 1999) identified certain factors that could hinder the use of alternative postures for delivery, such as the power and control over decision-making that doctors hold in the clinical area. Midwives had little or no opportunity to encourage women to use the upright postures for labour or delivery. Moreover, most deliveries in Singapore were performed by doctors, and midwives were not empowered to be autonomous. The study found that some midwives in the UK appeared reluctant to use the upright posture because of their ambivalent attitude towards it. Walsh (2000) argues that this must be because the majority of normal births following low intervention labours occur with women in the semi-recumbent or supine position.

In addition, four main studies (Hanson, 1998a, 1998b; Walsh, 1998; Walsh et al, 1999) found that changing practice attitude towards the move from recumbent, supine or lithotomy position to upright postures can succeed through re-education. On the other hand, the high interventionist approach to care within a hospital environment can prevent women from delivering in the upright position (Coppen, 1999). These findings suggest that, no matter how hard one tries to re-educate midwives, there are significant factors beyond the midwives' control that hinder their progress.

Perhaps it is time to re-focus these objectives away from the midwives and onto the women in their care. There is a need to re-educate women in the antenatal period, to empower and encourage them to use the upright position for labour and delivery. The need to return control to the women and reinforce the choices available to them is vital in the present climate of an interventionist and medicalised approach to midwifery care. The challenge for midwives is to change their attitudes and practice and focus on the women in their care by re-educating them about the benefits of the upright posture for delivery.

Conclusion

The review highlights the importance of informing and educating women about birthing positions to empower them to make a decision based on the evidence for the use of the upright position in childbirth. It concludes that lack of knowledge and autonomy on the part of the midwife has played a role in the continuing trend towards the use of recumbent positions in current practice, and suggests that a deficit of information in the antenatal period on the benefits of the upright posture may have hindered its use during childbirth. The NHS Centre for Reviews and Dissemination supported a study on giving women informed choice and produced several leaflets on various pregnancy-related topics, including positions in labour and delivery (MIDIRS 1996, 2003). However, the value of the leaflets has not been fully evaluated.

The present review begs several questions:

1. Is there a need to increase women's knowledge and decision-making skills in relation to choice perception concerning upright positions for childbirth?
2. Is there evidence to show that women are aware of the different choices of birthing positions available to them?
3. Is there evidence to show that women prefer to use the upright position in childbirth?
4. How clear is the evidence favouring upright positions over recumbent positions?

With regard to questions 1 and 2, the review has identified gaps in the literature resulting from an absence of research on choice and the decision-making process concerning positions in labour.

With regard to question 3, the review affirms that women do have a preference regarding birthing positions. Evidence in favour of the upright posture was apparent in historical (88%), comparative (80%) and descriptive (92%) studies, and in six non-systematic reviews (67%), including empirical evidence from 16 (64%) randomised controlled trials, 5 (74%) quasi-experimental studies and 1 (50%) prospective cohort study.

The evidence in this review indicates that most women prefer the upright position for childbirth, mainly from previous experience of it or from having a negative experience with the recumbent position. This suggests that women lack the necessary knowledge to choose the position that would best meet their individual needs, thus highlighting a lack of choice perception and indicating a need for further research on birthing positions.

A lack of empirical research concerning the value of education in increasing women's knowledge and enhancing their choice of birthing position is evident from this review. The review therefore provides the rationale for conducting a randomised controlled trial to compare the value of existing approaches to educating women with that of an innovative approach (provision of focused information) in enhancing women's knowledge levels and decision-making. The results of such studies would be invaluable in changing current practice, where the information given may be inaccurate and not evidence based. By highlighting women's preferred birthing positions, the findings might also encourage more women to adopt the upright position throughout the labour process, thereby enhancing their birth experience. The study will be in line with government proposals on keeping women informed about their choices in all aspects of maternity care (Department of Health, 1993; MIDIRS, 1996; Department of Health, 1997; MIDIRS, 2003; WHO, 1999; Department of Health, 2004, 2005).

It was also important to obtain midwives' views of birthing positions and to determine whether midwives know what is best for women in labour, or whether women know what is best for them and want midwives to accommodate their wishes. The results of a survey of a cohort of midwives, discussed in Section II, may provide the answers.

Overall, the results of the systematic literature review provided sufficient evidence in support of the hypothesis that there are benefits to be gained from adopting the upright posture in childbirth, and that, given the choice, women would choose the upright position. Gaps in the literature concerning women and midwives' decision-making processes in relation to birthing positions have been highlighted.

In light of the review, it was hypothesised that the provision of focused information, as a strategy to enhance knowledge, reduce decisional conflict and encourage women to adopt the upright posture in childbirth, will empower women in their decision-making. The challenge for the researcher (the author) was to develop a strategy to assist women in making their choices and preferences known to the midwives, and to find out what women want in relation to birthing positions. The results of the randomised controlled trial conducted by the author to test this hypothesis are presented in Chapters 8 and 9. The discussion and conclusion will follow in Chapter 10.

Section 11

Section II

CHAPTER 6

Midwives' views on birthing positions

To understand why recumbent positions are still in common use in midwifery practice today, it is important to determine the views and preferences of professional midwives regarding the birthing positions they would use to deliver the women in their care. In so doing, we may discover the rationale for this practice and highlight circumstances where midwives would or would not deliver in the upright position. The results of the study presented here will provide a greater understanding of midwives' attitudes and behaviour towards the use of different positions, which may in turn improve the quality of care provided to women during childbirth.

A systematic review of the literature on midwives' views of birthing positions found a dearth of publications on this topic. Only seven studies were found that had attempted to survey midwives' views of birthing positions (Clements, 1994; Coppen, 1997; Hanson, 1998a, 1998b; Walsh, 1998; Walsh et al, 1999; Coppen, 1999).

Hanson (1998a, 1998b) surveyed 800 midwives about their practice with regard to birthing positions, particularly the lithotomy position. The results showed that 60% of women were delivered in a non-lithotomy position. Three midwives indicated that they used the lithotomy position exclusively because it was what they were used to and were experienced with.

Walsh (1998) conducted an exploratory study with 40 midwives to determine the effectiveness of evidence-based information on the benefits of using alternative positions. The midwives attended an active birth workshop followed by weekly forum sessions to promote the use of upright positions. There was a dramatic change in the use of upright postures – from 18% to 46% – in the first 3 months following the exposure. Midwives' preferences regarding birthing positions were: kneeling (29%), all fours (28%) and left lateral (23%). This study provided evidence that changing practice attitudes towards a move from recumbent, supine or lithotomy positions to upright postures can succeed through re-education. However, it is not known how long midwives would continue this trend, or whether it was merely due to the Hawthorne effect. An audit of midwifery birthing practice in the following year (Walsh et al, 1999) showed that the use of upright postures had levelled out at 43%, suggesting that re-education had played a role in influencing midwifery practice in this group of midwives; however, it was not clear whether the same group of 40 midwives were involved in the audit.

A focus group of 10 midwives from a large teaching hospital in London were asked their views on the use of alternative birthing positions (Coppen, 1997). Eight of the 10 midwives (80%) indicated that they were willing to deliver women in the upright posture. The midwives would suggest an alternative position to the woman if labour was not progressing well. A common theme in this study was that although a woman may choose an upright position, the advent of compulsory monitoring of the woman, induction of labour and pressure from the obstetrician may prevent the midwives from encouraging its use. The study also revealed that while an alternative position is considered an option for the women, it is not the norm.

In a small comparative study (Coppen, 1999), 75 midwives (36 from the UK, 39 from Singapore) were asked their views and knowledge of eight different birthing positions before and after attending a seminar on birthing positions. The midwives' knowledge base increased following the seminar workshop, although the increase in the Singapore group was less that that in the UK group. The study also found that Singapore midwives were less exposed to delivering women in the upright posture. This was attributed to three main factors: lack of opportunity, not being empowered to do so by the obstetrician and not being educated about the advantages of upright postures for delivery. The same group of midwives also perceived that women prefer to lie down on the bed throughout labour. In contrast, British midwives had more opportunity and ability to deliver women in the upright posture. This study highlighted the need for further research to determine whether midwives were able to use their increased knowledge base in the clinical setting.

The question of whether midwives prefer one birthing position over another, however, and the rationale for their choices have not been investigated. This gap in the literature prompted the author to undertake the research study presented in this chapter. The entire population of midwives from one clinical setting, with different midwifery backgrounds, length of experience and ages, were included in the study to ensure that a representative sample of midwives' views was obtained. The aim was to gain a better understanding of midwives' attitudes towards the use of different positions.

Methods

Ethical approval

The Divisional Research Ethics Committee in Mid-Surrey approved the study in March 2000. The nature of the survey and the data collection method were explained in full to the committee, who were also informed of an earlier study undertaken to test the validity and reliability of the questionnaire that would be used to collect the data from the midwives.

The survey questionnaire

A questionnaire to determine midwives' preferences and views of nine different birthing positions, and to assess their attitude and hence their reasons for their highest and lowest preference scores, was developed for the survey (*Appendix 5*). The development of the questionnaire was influenced by a small focus group study (Coppen, 1997) conducted on a group of midwives to determine their views of birthing positions. The questionnaire was piloted on a group of midwives in a London teaching hospital in 1999 and any ambiguity was addressed and clarified in readiness for the midwives in this study (Coppen, 1999).

Internal validity and repeatability of the questionnaire were assessed using Pearson's correlation coefficient. Pearson's coefficient is calculated when two variables are measured on at least the interval scale, and is a descriptive and inferential statistical test. As a descriptive statistic, it summarises the magnitude and direction of a relationship between two variables (Polit and Hungler, 1999). Pearson's correlation coefficient using bivariate analysis for the nine different birthing positions was considered significant at $P<0.01$. Test-retest of the questionnaire on 10 midwives from another clinical site confirmed that the questionnaire was a reliable measure of what it purported to measure.

The questionnaire consisted of 12 questions designed to elicit midwives' views of nine different birthing positions. For simplicity, visual analogue scales and tick boxes were used to identify the midwives' preferences.

The main thrust of the questionnaire was to obtain midwives' preferences from nine different positions in such a way that they could be quantified. Midwives were asked to identify their preference for one type of position over another based on nine possible delivery positions: recumbent, semi-recumbent, left lateral, lithotomy, squatting, semi-squatting, kneeling, all-fours and standing positions. The lithotomy position was included as there is evidence that some midwives are still delivering women in this position (Coppen, 1994; Hanson 1998a, 1998b). The midwives were then asked to rate their preferences on a scale of 0–100%, giving the lowest score to the weakest preference and the highest score to the strongest preference.

The midwives were also asked to state their reasons for their choice of most preferred and least preferred positions.

Sampling

The questionnaire included demographic details (age, working hours, length of experience, place of work and duration of clinical allocation) of the midwives in the survey. This survey method requires respondents to be a representative sample of the population from which they were drawn, in order to obtain objective data for statistical analysis. The midwives surveyed worked in a small unit with a delivery rate of just over 2000 per year. The full complement of midwives working in this unit was 80. Following discussion with the statistician, it was decided that all the midwives, including 21 bank midwives on the payroll and two regular agency staff (i.e. on the payroll at least once a week), should be included in the survey to ensure full representation.

Study procedure

Following ethical approval, the researcher wrote to all the midwives in the unit to be surveyed, informing them of the purpose of the study and inviting them to complete the enclosed questionnaire, and to obtain their consent. An information sheet was also enclosed, inviting them to a seminar to be held in the unit following completion of the questionnaire. A poster of the study to be conducted in the unit was distributed to all the midwifery sites. The midwives were also informed that confidentiality would be maintained at all times and that they were under no obligation to complete the questionnaire. Consent was implied through completion of the questionnaire.

They were asked to return the questionnaire in purpose-built boxes, which were placed at three sites – the antenatal clinic, delivery suite and community midwife's office within the maternity unit – for the convenience of the midwives and to reduce the cost of posting.

Response rate

Of the 80 questionnaires sent out, 62 were returned within 2 weeks. Eighteen reminders were sent to the midwives who were yet to complete the questionnaire. Of these, five were returned (including one that was blank), giving a total of 66 completed questionnaires. There were 12 non-responders, whose age group and staff grade were evenly distributed across the range. Of these, six were bank midwives and two were midwives employed by the NHS. A further two midwives had moved house and two had recently left their place of work. There were no significant differences between responders and non-responders in relation to age, clinical allocation, employment grade and total number of working hours. There was one form missing from a midwife who was working part-time in education and part-time in the community.

It is important to know as much as possible about non-responders as they may have different characteristics from responders (Moser and Kalton, 1971). However, it could also be argued that it is unethical to approach non-responders, as by declining to participate they have not given their consent for the use of their data (Wagstaff, 2000). To overcome this problem, basic characteristics of the non-responding midwives, such as age, area of work and years of experience, were obtained from the midwifery manager. The data were matched against those of responders with similar characteristics. This meant that the coding system of identifying the midwives had to be used. However, to reduce researcher bias, this was not done until after completion of the analysis.

Overall, 67 of the 80 questionnaires sent out were returned, giving an excellent response rate of 84%. There is no agreement as to what constitutes an adequate response rate in survey research. Miller (1991) suggested that response rates for surveys are often low and that a 50% response rate may be obtained if the survey is conducted by an inexperienced person. Treece and Treece (1986) considered a response rate of 75–85% from a postal survey to be very good. Mason (1989) found that a low response rate is often obtained when those surveyed are from a minority group. Interestingly, most of the midwives in the survey were caucasian (91%).

Data analysis

Each completed questionnaire was coded and the data were entered into an Excel database and analysed using the SPSS statistical package. Inferential statistics were used to determine whether there was any causal relationship or correlation between the variables. Most of the data were analysed using non-parametric and chi-squared analysis, except for continuous variables such as age and years of experience, where parametric tests were used. Any correlation and association between respondents was then identified.

Qualitative data (open questions) were analysed using open coding (Glaser, 1992). Open coding is a process of breaking down and conceptualising the data (Holloway and Wheeler, 1996a). Hutchinson (1986) differentiates between three code levels. Level 1 codes are simple, e.g. a mother may comment 'my labour was very painful this time round'. The code for this might be 'painful labour'. It is very similar to latent content analysis, which involves categorising words and phrases with a conceptual label that describes them (Donovan, 2000). The words and phrases can be counted using a computer, to identify the frequency with which they appear. In this way, concepts and themes emerge from the data. Level 2 codes consist of concepts linked to form categories. For example, concepts related to use of the squatting position, such as 'too awkward', 'difficult to move' and 'hard to squat', form a category entitled 'problems with positions'. Further linking and reduction of the categories to form major categories produces level 3 codes, e.g. 'hindering factors'.

Codes may consist of words or phrases used by participants to describe a phenomenon identified by Strauss (1987) as 'in-vivo codes'. For example, a midwife in this survey commented 'I have not been taught to deliver in the upright posture'. The code might then be 'not been taught to deliver'. In-vivo codes can give life and interest to the study and are immediately recognised as reflecting the reality of the participants (Holloway and Wheeler, 1996a,b). Latent content analysis and in-vivo codes were used to analyse open-ended questions and comments and to identify themes in both the survey and the RCT.

Results

Of the 80 midwives sent questionnaires, 67 responded, giving a response rate of 84%. One returned a blank questionnaire, so the results presented here are based on the responses from 66 midwives. Where appropriate, the chi-squared differences in results between age groups are shown. This is reflected by the different totals at the end of the columns in some of the tables.

There were no significant differences in the distribution of grades between the age groups 25–36 years and 37–48 years *(Table 6.1)*. However, there was a significant difference (P<0.01) in the distribution of senior grades between the 25–36 years age group and the 49–60 years age group: the G grade midwives were older and the majority of midwives at the two lower grades were in the younger age groups.

There were 20 (30%) G grade (sister level) midwives, of whom 11 worked full time and 9 part time. Almost half the midwives (30; 45%) were employed at F grade (junior sister): seven of these worked full time and 23 part time. Midwives employed at E grade (staff midwife) formed the smallest group (16; 24%). The majority of these worked part time; this was because most were also bank midwives, and two were agency midwives.

TABLE 6.1: Distribution of grades by age group

Age group	Grade G	Grade F	Grade E	Total
25–36 years	3	11	9	23
37–48 years	8	14	5	27
49–60 years	9	5	2	16
TOTAL	20	30	16	66

Chi-squared = 9.358, P<0.01, 2df Significant

TABLE 6.2: Distribution of grades and whole-time equivalents

Grade	Full time	Part time	Total
G	11	9	20
F	7	23	30
E	3	11	14
Agency	0	2	2
TOTAL	21	45	66

TABLE 6.3: Distribution of full-time and part-time staff by grade

Age group	Grade G	Grade F	Grade E	Total
Full time	11	7	3	21
Part time	9	23	11	43
TOTAL	20	30	14	64

Chi-squared = 6.512, P<0.05, 2df Significant

Table 6.2 shows the distribution of staff by grade and whether they worked part time or full time. In total, 45 (68%) midwives worked part time and 21 (32%) worked full time.

Excluding the two agency midwives, the difference between the number of full-time and part-time staff at each grade was significant (P<0.05) (*Table 6.3*).

Midwives were asked about their main clinical allocation. *Figure 6.1* shows that the greatest proportion of the midwives (25; 38%) worked in the delivery suite, followed by community placement (19; 29%) and rotation (12; 18%), which meant that midwives worked between wards. The emphasis placed on delivery suite allocation is clearly demonstrated.

Midwives were also asked how long they had been working at their particular clinical allocation. *Figure 6.2* shows that almost a third of the midwives (21; 32%) had worked in the delivery suite for 5 years or more.

The majority of midwives (52%) had more than 10 years' experience. The second largest group (15%) had 8–10 years' experience. Only two midwives had less than one year's experience (*Table 6.4*). There was a stepwise increase in midwives' length of experience when plotted against the number of midwives (*Figure 6.3*), contrasting the lowest number of midwives, who had the least experience, and the highest number, with the most experience.

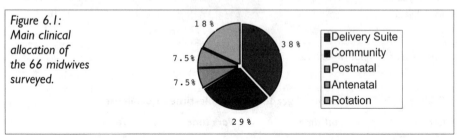

Figure 6.1:
Main clinical
allocation of
the 66 midwives
surveyed.

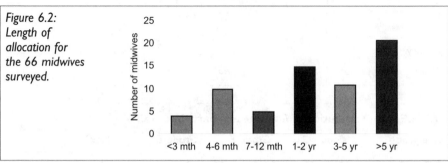

Figure 6.2:
Length of
allocation for
the 66 midwives
surveyed.

TABLE 6.4: Length of experience as a midwife

Length of experience	No. of midwives (%)
<1 year	2 (3%)
1–2 years	5 (8%)
3–4 years	7 (11%)
5–7 years	8 (12%)
8–10 years	10 (15%)
>10 years	34 (52%)
TOTAL	66 (100%)

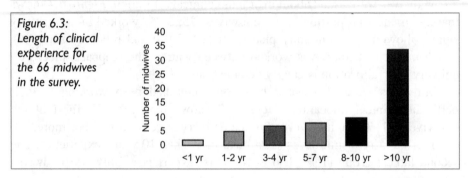

Figure 6.3:
Length of clinical
experience for
the 66 midwives
in the survey.

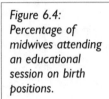

Figure 6.4:
Percentage of
midwives attending
an educational
session on birth
positions.

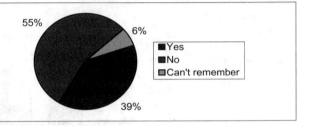

The number of midwives who had attended an educational session on birthing positions was surprisingly low: 26 (39%) had attended *vs* 36 (55%) who had not attended (*Figure 6.4*). The majority of those who had not attended an educational session had 8 or more years' experience.

The midwives' preferences for one type of position over another are summarised in *Table 6.5*. The differences in the totals show that some midwives did not respond to this question or left some of the preferences out. However, the differences are small and do not affect the overall results. Overall, 38 (58%) midwives had a strong or very strong preference for the all-fours position, and 35 (53%) a strong or very strong preference for the semi-recumbent position and the kneeling position. Slightly more midwives had a very strong preference for the semi-recumbent position. Of those who identified a strong or very strong preference for the semi-recumbent position, 32 (91%) were more experienced midwives with 8 or more years' experience. Ranking third in this category was the left lateral position (33; 51%). The majority of the midwives (57; 92%) indicated a very weak to weak preference for the recumbent position, closely followed by the lithotomy position (51; 82%) and the standing position (35; 55%). Surprisingly, three midwives (5%) indicated a strong or very strong preference for the recumbent and lithotomy positions.

TABLE 6.5: Midwives' preferences for a particular delivery position

	Very weak	Weak	Neutral	Strong	Very strong	Total responses
Recumbent	55	2	2	3	0	62
Semi-recumbent	6	8	17	9	26	66
Left lateral	9	11	12	15	18	65
Lithotomy	40	11	8	2	1	62
All-fours (hands & knees)	4	6	17	17	21	65
Squatting	10	17	16	10	8	61
Semi-squatting	9	11	18	11	11	60
Standing	16	19	15	7	7	64
Kneeling	7	7	16	13	22	65

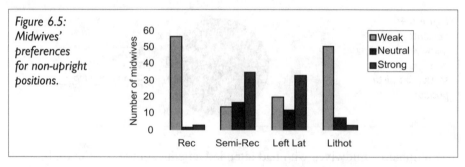

Figure 6.5:
Midwives'
preferences
for non-upright
positions.

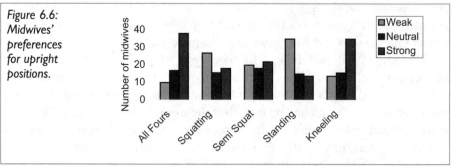

Figure 6.6:
Midwives'
preferences
for upright
positions.

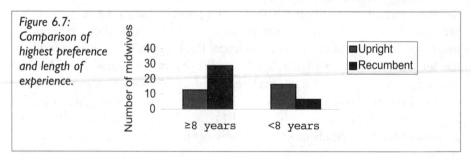

Figure 6.7:
Comparison of
highest preference
and length of
experience.

Figure 6.5 shows midwives' preferences for non-upright positions (recumbent, semi-recumbent, left lateral and lithotomy), with the data combined into three categories (very weak and weak preferences; neutral preference; strong and very strong preferences). Semi-recumbent and left lateral positions show similar patterns, with the weakest preference for recumbent and lithotomy positions.

Figure 6.6 shows midwives' preferences for upright positions (all-fours, squatting, semi-squatting, standing and kneeling). The all-fours and kneeling positions scored the highest preference, with 38 midwives and 35 midwives respectively rating it their strong or very strong preference.

Figure 6.7 compares midwives' highest preferences for recumbent or upright positions with their years of experience. A significant association was found between midwives' years of experience and their highest preference for a particular position group (chi-squared 8.255, P<0.005, 1 df).

Midwives were also asked to give the reasons for their most preferred position. All the midwives in the survey responded to this question. The midwives' comments provide a rich source of data on their rationale for their most preferred position. Following content analysis of the data, and in-vivo coding, five core themes emerged: comfort for the women; familiarity with the position; women's choice/control; physical advantage for the women; and physical agility and accessibility for the midwife (*Table 6.6*). The frequency of occurrence of each theme is shown in the second column in *Table 6.6*.

TABLE 6.6: Thematic analysis of midwives' choice of position and frequency of occurrence

Core themes	Frequency of occurrence
Comfortable for the women	20
Familiarity with the position	8
Women's choice/control	13
Physical advantage for the women	40
Physical agility and accessibility for the midwife	16

Examples of how initial phrases or words were combined to form the core themes are shown in *Table 6.7*.

It is interesting to note that the need to be in control of the delivery was highlighted by those midwives who identified recumbent positions as their highest preference. Their comments included:

> *'It is the best position with CTG'*
> *'It is best for the midwife to see and control delivery of the head'*
> *'Access to the perineum and control of the head'*
> *'I am most confident with it and easier to control the head'*
> *'Good view and control of the perineum'*
> *'Easier to see, cleaner and better for back'*

By contrast, the need to give women control over the delivery was highlighted by those midwives who chose upright positions as their highest preference. Their comments included:

> *'Mothers seem to be more in control'*
> *'Gravity, maximum pelvic outlet and woman is in control'*
> *'Easier to push and women more in control'*
> *'Mobility for women and easier to push'*
> *'Woman copes well and can control her own pushing'*

TABLE 6.7: Words or phrases used by midwives

Words or phrases	Core themes
Most mothers feel comfortable; more comfortable for the mother; it was comfortable and acceptable for the mother; whatever is comfortable for the client; easier and more comfortable for women to adopt (recumbent)	Comfortable for the women
It is the one I have been most familiar with; certain position is adapted to situation; most common position taught during training; midwife's own experience (recumbent)	Familiarity with the position
Most patients choose for themselves; women's preferences; woman's choice; women more in control; allow women to deliver in the position they most prefer (mixture of recumbent/upright)	Women's choice/control
Gravity aids progress; optimisation of pelvic perineum; increases outlet and use of gravity; good utero-placental perfusion (upright)	Physical advantage for the women
Good visual and physical access for the midwife; accessible for midwife to view the perineum; good visibility of the perineum: less strain on midwife; the whole perineum is visible; better view of fetal head and perineum (recumbent)	Physical agility and accessibility for the midwife

Brackets indicate whether midwives were referring to the upright or recumbent position as their highest preference

The dichotomy within the themes, as the 'pieces of jigsaw' unfolded between midwives who were in favour of recumbent positions and those who favoured the upright position, is summarised in *Figure 6.8*. Four opposing themes emerged, as shown in each jigsaw, between recumbent and upright postures. In the first jigsaw, midwives identified that they preferred the recumbent position because it was comfortable for them and they were in control. At the same time, they also acknowledged the disadvantages of the recumbent position, highlighting

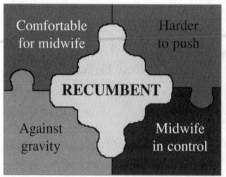 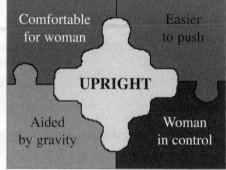

Figure 6.8: Dichotomy jigsaw for the recumbent and upright positions.

that this was an awkward position, which made it harder for the women to push during the second stage as they were pushing against the force of gravity. By contrast, in the second jigsaw, midwives who preferred the upright position identified that they were more able to focus on the women and acknowledged that it was more comfortable for the women and the women were more in control of the childbirth process. Midwives also highlighted that maintaining the upright position made it easier for the women to push, aided by the force of gravity.

Midwives were asked to identify to what extent they would be willing to deliver in a position they were not experienced with while caring for a woman in labour. The results are shown in *Table 6.8*.

TABLE 6.8: Willingness to deliver in a particular position at woman's request although inexperienced in its use

How willing?	Number (%)
Yes, definitely	30 (45%)
Yes, possibly	34 (52%)
No	2 (3%)
Total no. of responses = 66	

Most midwives (97%) responded positively to meeting a woman's request for a particular position, despite not having the experience: 45% were definite and 52% were possibly certain to meet the woman's request. Only two midwives said they were unwilling to deliver in a position with which they were not experienced, regardless of the woman's request.

Midwives were also asked if they would deliver a woman in a position that they were experienced with but did not feel comfortable with. There were five possible responses for them to choose from, as shown in *Table 6.9*. Only 5% of midwives indicated that they would not be willing; the majority again responded positively to this question, with 37% responding definitely and 58% saying 'yes, possibly'.

TABLE 6.9: Willingness to deliver in a position that you are experienced with but do not feel comfortable using

How willing?	Number (%)
Yes, definitely	24 (37%)
Yes, possibly	37 (58%)
No, but may give in to pressure by the women	3 (5%)
No, but may give in to peer pressure	0
Definitely not, regardless of the woman's wishes	0
Total no. of responses = 64	

In the penultimate section of the questionnaire, midwives were asked if they could describe, in their professional opinion, why most women deliver their baby on the bed in the recumbent or semi-recumbent position. All but one of the midwives (65; 98%) responded to this question, and 130 different reasons were given. On average, each midwife identified 2.0 separate issues. Content analysis of the comments highlighted six main themes that may have resulted in the current practice regarding the use of recumbent and semi-recumbent positions. These were:

º   Traditional influence/bed as focus
º   Midwife's influence
º   Media/friends' influence
º   Lack of education/information
º   Use of analgesia/monitors
º   Women's expectation.

The frequency with which these reasons were cited by the midwives is summarised in *Table 6.10*. It can be seen that midwives perceived that the women's expectation of using the recumbent or semi-recumbent position ranked highest, being cited no less than 42 times.

TABLE 6.10: Thematic analysis of midwives' views of the practice norm regarding the use of recumbent and semi-recumbent positions

Themes	Frequency of occurrence
Traditional influence/bed as focus	29
Midwife's influence	22
Media/friends' influence	12
Lack of education/awareness	15
Use of analgesia/monitor	10
Women's expectation	42
Total number of responses =130	

Traditional influence and/or bed as a focus received the second highest ranking, being mentioned no less than 32 times by 73% of midwives with 8 or more years' experience. Interestingly, it was the experienced midwives who indicated a preference for the recumbent positions. The midwife's influence on women's choice of birthing positions was also highlighted, being mentioned 22 times.

Some of the midwives' comments for each theme are reproduced below, in order of frequency, starting with the highest frequency:

1. Women's expectation

'Women expect to deliver in this position and when asked to change they seem surprised!'
'Women find it most comfortable'
'Women's choice, tiredness and more support from the bed'
'Women's perception of acceptable delivery position'
'Women are usually tired at this stage and do not have the energy to change'
'Women's need to remain in control'
'Most mothers appear comfortable in this position'
'Acceptable positions for comfort'

2. Traditional influence/bed as focus

'Tradition and seen as acceptable'
'Tradition due to socialisation and cultural issues'
'Bed is the focus in the delivery room, women feel they have to use it'
'Tradition and bed is the focus in the delivery suite compared to home-births, which are less inhibiting'
'Bed is the focus'
'Tradition! It is a habit'

3. Midwife's influence

'Suggestion of the midwife'
'Staff put mothers in bed compared with home-births'
'Midwives with bad back actually choose the semi-recumbent position to prevent further damage'
'Midwives do not discuss alternative positions with them'
'Midwives/doctors are used to it'
'Easy access for midwife to see the perineum'
'Midwives' lack of experience'

4. Lack of education/awareness

'Women believe it is the way to deliver due to lack of education'
'Most students are trained in this method'
'I was taught in this way and it is one of the most comfortable positions for them'
'No options given to mother, uninformed'
'Women don't know there are other positions'
'Lack of knowledge of alternative positions may play a part'
'Not given alternative by staff'

'*Mothers are not aware of the benefits of delivering in the alternative position*'

5. Media/friends' influence

'*Television personalities delivering in this way*'
'*Media influences*'
'*Influence by previous mothers in birthing position*'
'*Media and cultural influences*'
'*Influence of friends*'
'*Television influence*'
'*What they see in books and magazines*'

6. Use of analgesia/monitors

'*Increased demand for epidural*'
'*Monitoring, IV infusion, tiredness and mattresses not on the floor*'
'*Analgesia which makes more active position too tiring*'
'*Epidural analgesia*'
'*Attach to monitors and CTG*' and '*Easier for CTG*'

Finally, midwives were asked which professional journals they read regularly. The purpose of this question was to determine whether regular reading of professional journals correlated with a midwife's preference for a particular type of birthing position.

Sixty-four (97%) of the 66 midwives surveyed responded to this question; two left it blank. Responses showed that 34 (53%) midwives regularly read the MIDIRS journal *Midwifery Digest*, but the highest read journal was the *Royal College of Midwives (RCM) Midwives Journal*, which was read by 40 (63%) midwives. The *British Journal of Midwifery* (BJM) was read by only 16 (24%) midwives and the least read journals were medical journals, such as *British Medical Journal* (BMJ) and the *British Journal of Obstetrics and Gynaecology* (BJOG), or *Midwifery Journal*, which was read by only 2 (3%) midwives.

Further analysis showed that 27 (42%) midwives read more than one journal, a quarter (16; 25%) read only the RCM journal, and 11 (17%) read the MIDIRS journal alone. In total, 14 (22%) read the MIDIRS or RCM journals, 4 (6%) read the MIDIRS journal and BJM regularly, and 6 (9%) read a combination of the RCM journal and BJM regularly. Nine (14%) midwives also read *The Practising Midwife* journal. Other less read midwifery journals were *Professional Nurse* (1), *Midwifery Matters* (2), *AIMS Journal* (1), *The Practitioner* (1), *The Register* (UKCC journal) (2). One midwife also cited the internet as a reading source. The four main journals read regularly by the cohort of midwives are shown in *Figure 6.9*.

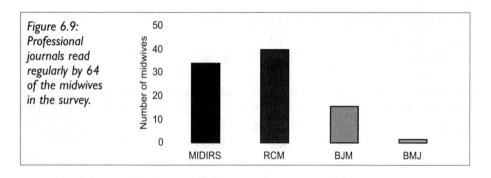

Figure 6.9:
Professional
journals read
regularly by 64
of the midwives
in the survey.

Overall, the midwives read three main journals regularly. The highest read journal was the *RCM Midwives Journal*, a monthly journal produced by the RCM and distributed free to all members. The second most read journal was the MIDIRS *Midwifery Digest*, a quarterly journal containing a selection of published research and non-research based studies from a wide range of sources; it claims to scan approximately 500 journals in the search for new information. It is a popular journal and one that educationalists often recommend to midwifery students and return-to-practice midwives because of its ability to access a variety of studies from peer-reviewed and popular journals both nationally and internationally. The third most read journal was the *British Journal of Midwifery*, a monthly journal, which is relatively new and was first published less than a decade ago.

The journals that midwives read the least were the medical journals, such as the *British Medical Journal* and the *Journal of Obstetrics and Gynaecology*, which were read by only two midwives. An analysis of the journals read regularly is shown in *Table 6.11*.

TABLE 6.11: Analysis of professional journals read regularly

Professional journal	No. of midwives (%)
RCM Midwives Journal only	16 (25%)
MIDIRS *Midwifery Digest* only	11 (17%)
British Journal of Midwifery only	4 (6%)
Combination of *RCM Midwives Journal* and MIDIRS journal	14 (22%)
Combination of *British Journal of Midwifery* and MIDIRS journal	4 (6%)
Combination of *RCM Midwives Journal* and *British Journal of Midwifery*	6 (9%)
Combination of *RCM Midwives Journal* or MIDIRS journal and *Practising Midwife* journal	9 (14%)
Combination of *Midwifery* and medical journal	2 (3%)
Three journals or more	9 (14%)

Of the 40 midwives who read the *RCM Midwives Journal*, 30 (75%) chose semi-recumbent or left lateral positions as their highest preference. Of the 38 midwives who read the MIDIRS journal regularly, 20 (53%) opted for the semi-recumbent or left lateral position as their highest preference; this group included at least two midwives who had a strong preference for the lithotomy position. By contrast, of the 14 midwives who also read the BJM, 10 (71%) chose an upright position as their highest preference. Interestingly, the only two midwives who read the *Midwifery* professional journal and a medical journal also chose the upright position as their highest preference. *Table 6.12* shows the contrast and association between journal(s) read and highest preference for delivery position in labour.

TABLE 6.12: Association between journal(s) read and highest preference for delivery position

No. of midwives (%)	Journals read	Recumbent position (no. %)
40 (61%)	RCM Midwives Journal	30 (75%)
38 (58%)	MIDIRS Midwifery Digest	20 (53%)
No. of midwives (%)	Journals read	Upright position (no. %)
14 (21%)	British Journal of Midwifery	10 (71%)
2 (3%)	Midwifery and medical	2 (100%)

These findings suggest that midwives who read the RCM or MIDIRS journal were more likely to select the semi-recumbent position or left lateral position as their highest preference. By contrast, midwives whose repertoire of read journals also included the BJM, *Midwifery* or a medical journal were more likely to choose an upright position as their highest preference.

Discussion of the findings

This study investigated midwives' views and preferences regarding the use of nine different delivery positions. Analysis of the midwives' age and grade of employment showed that the majority of midwives working in the maternity unit where the survey was undertaken were older and more experienced: 52% had more than 10 years' experience compared with only 22% with less than 4 years' experience. In addition, significantly more E and F grade midwives were employed as part-time staff than as full-time staff (P<0.05). These findings are not surprising in light of the current national recruitment problem

(Department of Health, 2001) and the emphasis on employers to take on part-time staff and introduce flexible working hours (Department of Health, 1998a, 2000). The results suggest that the unit where these midwives are employed recognises the need for a flexible and family-oriented approach to employment.

The findings also reveal that the majority (45%) of the senior G grade midwives within the age range 49–60 years had worked in this unit for more than 10 years. In addition, 44% of midwives employed at F grade were aged between 37 and 48 years. Overall, there were considerably more midwives (67%) with 8 or more years' experience than midwives with 2 years or less experience (11%). The results also revealed a stepwise increase in clinical experience when the midwives were grouped according to length of experience (*Table 6.4*). This reflects the success of recruitment and retention of staff in this particular unit.

The majority of the midwives' clinical allocation in the maternity unit was concentrated in the delivery suite (37%). By contrast, only 8% of midwives were allocated to the antenatal clinic and postnatal ward. The major distribution of midwives to the delivery suite reflects the high priority given to the delivery suite; not surprisingly, the postnatal unit was the lowest priority. It may be that, as the average length of postnatal stay for the mother and baby within postnatal units in the UK decreases (Bick, 2000b), it makes sense to reduce the number of midwives allocated to such units. However, this does not take into account the high level of care required by some mothers in the postnatal unit; it merely reflects the importance and immediate needs of the delivery suite.

A seminal work on workload measurement in midwifery (Ball, 1993) highlighted the emphasis on caring for women throughout labour and delivery. This would explain why high staffing levels are often needed in the delivery suite.

Surprisingly, only 26 (39%) midwives had attended an educational session on birth positions. It may be that the midwives lacked the opportunity to attend a session because of work overload or shortage of staff, or had never been given the opportunity to attend. Lack of opportunity to attend may reflect an element of restriction on attendance at professional updating sessions by midwives. This was apparent to the researcher when she organised six updating sessions as part of the requirements for ethical approval, and kept a detailed record in support of this discussion. Disappointingly, only nine of the midwives taking part in the survey attended. Some of the reasons given by the midwives for non-attendance are reproduced below:

'No time to attend'
'I wanted to attend but at the last minute was asked to stay on the unit'
'Not working in labour suite'
'Lack of staff in the unit'
'Had antenatal clinics to attend'

It is also possible that some midwives, especially those in a position to control which midwives may or may not attend, do not consider professional updating on birthing positions important enough to warrant time off. If this is the case, it is a cause for concern as midwives cannot be expected to practise evidence-based midwifery care if they are not aware of recent developments in research.

Robinson (1994) highlighted the problems of defining the relationship between provision of, and need for, continuing education and updating in a longitudinal study of midwives from two large cohorts – one comprising 932 midwives who qualified in 1979 after completing a 12-month course, and the other consisting of 931 midwives who qualified in 1983 after an 18-month course. Robinson found that those midwives who were obliged to undertake continuing education did not achieve as much as those who were motivated to attend. In addition, less than half the respondents had undertaken in-service training. This was attributed in part to lack of provision. Moreover, the two most common in-service training courses were those on management and parentcraft issues, yet the most desired education, highlighted as important by the midwives, was clinical updating.

Thus, in relation to poor attendance at the in-service training in the present study, it is reasonable to assume that those midwives who were taught to deliver only in the recumbent position 10–20 years ago will continue to do so if they are not aware of current evidence. In contrast, midwives who have been educated recently would have been taught the evidence for and against the use of recumbent *vs* upright positions, and will therefore be more more likely to apply that knowledge in their practice.

Indeed, the significant association found between the most experienced midwives, who opted for a recumbent position, and the less experienced midwives, who opted for an upright position, suggest that there may be some degree of complacency or lack of awareness among the experienced midwives with regard to evidence-based practice. This is a worrying prospect for student midwives and newly qualified midwives today, as many could be prevented from gaining the necessary experience needed to deliver women in the upright position if their senior colleagues were not up to date with current knowledge. They would be more likely to deliver in a position with which they are experienced and familiar. This may explain the continuing trend in the use of recumbent positions today. In addition, the findings on the lack of education on the use of different birthing positions provide some evidence to explain the current practice norms of using recumbent positions. However, this survey did not identify the extent of the midwives' knowledge of birthing positions – merely whether or not they had attended an educational session on the topic.

For the first time in a research study, midwives have been asked to identify their preferences from nine possible birthing positions. Previous studies

(Coppen, 1997; Hanson 1998a, 1998b; Walsh, 1998; Walsh et al, 1999) on this subject had sought to determine midwives views' on birthing positions in general, but had not asked them specifically about their preference for each of the nine positions outlined in this survey. A comparative study by Coppen (1999) did ask midwives from Singapore and the UK in what positions they normally delivered a baby, based on nine possible options. However, the study did not specifically ask midwives to rate their preferences for one type of position over another.

The findings in this survey on midwife's preferences from nine birthing positions found that 38 (58%) midwives had a strong or very strong preference for the all-fours position. The second highest preference was for the semi-recumbent position (41%), and then the kneeling position (33%), with 35 (53%) midwives opting for both positions. Surprisingly, at least 5% of midwives indicated a strong or very strong preference for the recumbent or lithotomy position.

Yet there is unequivocal evidence that recumbent and lithotomy birthing positions do not confer any benefits on the mother or baby (Diaz et al, 1980; Hemminki et al, 1986; Sleep et al, 1989; Gardosi et al, 1989b; De Jong et al, 1997; Larson, 1997; Shermer and Raines, 1997; Henty, 1998; Gupta and Nikodem, 2000a; Gupta and Hofmeyr, 2004). Dundes' (1987) explorative study of dorsal and lithotomy positions found that the adoption and use of lithotomy positions was not based on sound scientific evidence, and the birthing position was influenced by the interprofessional struggle between surgeons and midwives. The high preference for the semi-recumbent position suggests that, despite evidence contraindicating the use of this posture, midwives are reluctant to change their practice. Moreover, Thomson (1988), in her review of the literature on management of the second stage of labour more than a decade ago, questioned 'current' policies, which required women to deliver in the semi-recumbent or dorsal position. Current practice suggests that many midwives would offer women the option to deliver in the upright posture if women request it, which suggests that they may not necessarily promote its use either (Coppen, 2002). Therefore, it is not surprising that women are still delivering in the recumbent and semi-recumbent positions today (Coppen, 1994, Audit Commission, 1997; Garcia et al, 1996; Hanson, 1998a; Walsh, 1998; Coppen, 1999; Coppen, 2002; De Jonge and Lagro-Janssen, 2004; De Jonge et al, 2004).

More worrying is the fact that, in the present study, it was the experienced midwives who preferred to use the semi-recumbent position and the same group of 'experienced' midwives who had not attended an educational session on positions in labour. This suggests that the midwives were not aware of current evidence-based research on the use of upright positions. Perhaps the daily routine and policies in the labour ward are stifling midwives' autonomy and creative judgement (Garcia et al, 1986).

Current guidance recommends that women be given the option to deliver in whichever position they choose (Clinical Standards Advisory Group, 1995; NHS Centre for Reviews and Dissemination, 1996; Coppen, 2002; De Jonge and Lagro-Janssen, 2004; De Jonge et al, 2004).

However, whether the choice would be acceptable to the midwife caring for the woman during childbirth is questionable. It is reassuring to note that more midwives indicated a preference to deliver in the all-fours position (58%) compared with the semi-recumbent position (53%), although the differences were very small. The kneeling position featured high in the preference ranking, with 35 (53%) midwives indicating a strong or very strong preference for it. The use of the left lateral position ranked third in the preference ranking, with half the midwives (33; 50%) indicating a strong or very strong preference for it.

Use of the left lateral position dates back a long way – to Porteus (1892), who advocated it on the grounds of ease for the accoucheur and the position that preserved the woman's dignity. A study of 201 mothers in 1985 (Logue, 1991) found that the left lateral position increased the incidence of delivering with an intact perineum: 117 (58%) women in the left lateral position *vs* 33% in the dorsal position (P<0.0001).

Shorten et al (2002) also found that the lateral position was associated with the highest rate of intact perineum (66%), compared with 42% for the squatting position, especially for women having their first baby. The fact that half the midwives had a strong preference for using the left lateral position may reflect the importance they place on preservation of the woman's perineum, albeit at the expense of a longer labour. Keeping the perineum intact during childbirth is an important skill; it may be that, for some midwives, delivering in the left lateral position is the best method of optimising that skill.

In a review of alternative positions, Roberts (1980) found that the lateral and all-fours positions afforded more comfort for the mother and convenience for the midwife. Hanson (1998a) also found that most midwives used the semi-recumbent and left lateral positions in the second stage of labour. It may be that midwives are more comfortable using a position they are familiar with, and are therefore more likely to use it in their practice. It can be argued that no amount of evidence-based research could persuade a midwife to deliver a woman in the upright position unless she/he is given the opportunity to use it, has been educated in its use and has additional support from a more experienced midwife. However, this is unlikely to occur in the present climate of poor staffing levels and overworked staff (Davis, 2002), which was evident from this survey.

Five core themes emerged from analysis of the midwives' comments about their reasons for their most preferred position. Midwives who indicated a high preference for recumbent positions (which included semi-recumbent, lithotomy and left lateral positions) said it was because it was a comfortable position for the women. This reason was cited 20 times. Midwives also felt comfortable about using recumbent positions because they were familiar with them. This suggests that midwives who are unfamiliar with using upright positions would prefer not to deliver women in these positions.

Midwives who indicated a highest preference for the upright posture highlighted the need to give women choice and control over their decision to deliver in the upright posture. Some midwives commented that women would choose for themselves the position they most prefer. Interestingly, of the 40 (63%) midwives who preferred to use the upright posture, only 17 (26%) were able to identify its advantage in terms of aiding gravity. One midwife indicated that the use of the all-fours position 'allowed optimisation of the [pelvic] perineum' and that it was 'an easier position for the women to adopt'.

Conversely, midwives who indicated a high preference for the recumbent position identified the importance of having good physical access to the woman's perineum. The need for a better view of the perineum and that delivering in the recumbent position was more comfortable for their physical health, i.e. it would not worsen their backache, were also highlighted as important factors influencing the midwife's choice.

Analysis of all the midwives' comments revealed a 'dichotomy jigsaw' (*Figure 6.7*) in that midwives who chose the upright position as their highest preference were more in favour of providing comfort for the women and giving them control over their own body, whereas those who chose the recumbent positions were more concerned about their own physical needs and the importance of having control over the delivery. The concept of giving choice and control to the women was thus only apparent in midwives with a strong preference for upright positions. Their main philosophy appeared to be to empower women to take control of their birth, to facilitate their decision and preference for a particular birth position. By contrast, midwives who chose recumbent positions as their highest preference were less able to articulate the need to give women choice; instead, they emphasised the need to have control over the delivery.

The need for midwives to have control was also evident in responses to the question asking midwives to what extent they would be willing to adopt a position that they were not experienced with, at the woman's request. Only 46% of midwives indicated that they would definitely be willing to deliver in a particular position at the woman's request, even though they may not be experienced in its use. However, the majority (55%) were more tentative in their responses, which suggests that they were less willing to deliver a woman in a position if they were inexperienced in its use, regardless of the woman's request.

In order to evaluate the degree of flexibility in their attitude towards recumbent or upright positions, the midwives were asked whether they would still be willing to deliver a woman in a particular position if they were experienced in its use but not comfortable with it. Only 24 (38%) midwives were certain of doing so; the majority of midwives (37; 58%) indicated tentatively that they would possibly deliver a woman in a position with which they were not comfortable. Only three midwives said no, but indicated that they might give in to pressure by the women. It is reassuring that none of the midwives were totally opposed to delivering in a position that they were not comfortable with, at the woman's request. These findings suggest that midwives give women's needs greater priority than their own, with more than a third responding positively. However, there appears to be a degree of uncertainty, as indicated by the tentative responses from 58% of the midwives to using a position they were not comfortable with, but may possibly do so at the mother's request.

Midwives were then asked why, in their professional opinion, most women deliver their baby in the recumbent or semi-recumbent position. The purpose of this question was to identify whether midwives could give a reason for current practice norms. The majority of midwives (65; 98%) responded to this question. Content analysis revealed six main themes, which were measured against the frequency of citation by the midwives. The most frequent reason identified by the midwives was women's expectation. Many midwives felt that women expected to be in the recumbent positions because it was what they were used to. For example, one midwife said: 'Women expect to be in this position and when asked to change they seem surprised'.

Traditional practice was the second most common reason for present practice norms. For example, a midwife indicated that tradition due to socialisation and cultural issues has led to women delivering in the recumbent position. Some midwives commented that the bed as the focus in the delivery suite was also to blame for the common use of recumbent and semi-recumbent positions today.

The third theme in the ranking order was the midwife's influence. The honesty and integrity of the midwives who gave this as a reason is surpassed only by those who highlighted a lack of education and awareness as another reason why mothers continue to deliver in the recumbent positions. Several midwives commented that, because of a lack of education, some women believe that this is the way to deliver. Another said that most students are trained in this delivery position or were taught using this position and found it to be the most comfortable. If a lack of education is preventing women from delivering in the upright position, the need for all midwives to attend professional updating on the use of upright positions has never been greater or more urgent. Indeed, Walsh (1998) and Walsh et al (1999) showed that there were positive benefits to be gained from the midwife's attitude towards the use of the upright positions, once midwives had been re-educated and updated.

Several midwives commented that women's lack of education on the benefits of the upright position was a factor in their continuing use of recumbent positions for delivery. However, the findings also show that midwives themselves lacked the necessary education on the benefits of the upright position, which in turn led to the continued use of recumbent positions, especially semi-recumbent positions, during labour and delivery. Fenwick and Simkin (1987), McKay (1980), McKay (1984), Nelki and Bond (1995) and Nodine and Roberts (1987) highlighted the importance of education in informing women of the benefits of maternal movement and upright positioning during labour.

In previous studies, many mothers have indicated that they would like more information and knowledge about birthing positions so that they could make an informed decision or choice (Clements, 1994; Coppen, 1994; Gupta and Lilford, 1987; Housham, 1998). Yet parent education today is often piecemeal and many units do not focus on the use of upright birthing positions in antenatal classes. Instead, the philosophy is to provide a general education to women about care in labour as a whole.

The final question in this survey asked midwives which professional journals they read regularly. Studies have shown that midwives who read professional journals regularly are more up to date with evidence-based knowledge than those who do not (Hanson, 1998a, 1998b). This survey has shown that the majority of the midwives (63%) read the RCM journal regularly, and a quarter (25%) read only the RCM journal. Of these, only 20% indicated that they also read the MIDIRS journal regularly. Overall, just over a third (37%) read the MIDIRS journal regularly and only 1% of midwives were familiar with the medical journals.

These findings suggest that midwives whose only source of research awareness is derived from a basic journal that does not have a strong research ethos, rather than other internationally recognised journals such as *Midwifery*, BJM and BMJ, may not be keeping up to date with research-based knowledge. The reason for the lack of wide readership may be that midwives do not feel the need to read widely, or lack the time to read, or are simply not interested in reading any other professional journals. Or it may be that some midwives do not know how to access, or have difficulty in accessing, other journals.

A literature search found a limited number of studies on the effects of journal reading on evidence-based practice. Yeoh and Morrissey (1996) highlighted problems of accessing library facilities and resource availability in a survey of nurses, midwives and health visitors. They found that respondents required support for literature searching and accessing library facilities. It is therefore possible that the lack of journal readership in the midwives in the present survey was due to poor access to library facilities or a lack of resources to help midwives increase their knowledge. However, it is difficult to justify encouraging midwives to read more as there is only limited evidence that journal reading improves knowledge, hence it will have little influence in changing practice.

A study on the value of medical publications by Beasley (2000) was a critique on the proliferation of published papers. It proposed that there has been an explosion in medical publishing of doubtful and limited value. The author stated that good peer-reviewed journals are hard to find, and that a sudden increase in the quantity of journal publications on a particular topic does not necessarily mean an increase in quality. Beasley (2000) and Fletcher and Fletcher (1998) found that although the best articles on a particular topic tend to be concentrated in a few strong journals, good articles are scattered among different journals and a search of all the world's journals is required to find them.

To expect users to search the entire publication resource is both impractical and unnecessary. Searching the literature requires a certain element of skill, and a search of an inappropriate resource may be a waste of time and energy. Indeed, Soot et al (1999) found that 66% of medical information websites have virtually no useful information and some web pages have areas that are misleading or unrelated to the topic under investigation. Certainly, it is difficult to imagine that any practising midwives would have the time or the enthusiasm to search the literature either manually or via websites, except for a few who may need to survey all the essential literature in search of quality papers for research purposes. In addition, Hundley et al (2000) identified a number of barriers to midwives reading research articles: they had to do it in their own time; difficulties in accessing the library facilities; and lack of perceived value of research to practice. This may account for the lack of interest in reading more advanced research journals shown by midwives in the present survey.

Conclusion

The unit where the survey was undertaken was staffed mainly by older and experienced midwives. But despite this, only a third of the midwives had attended an educational session on birthing positions. The majority of the midwives were allocated to the delivery suite. More than half of the midwives had a strong or very strong preference for delivery in the semi-recumbent position, and the majority of these were experienced midwives. Over half the midwives had a strong or very strong preference for using the all-fours and kneeling positions and 50% had a strong preference for delivering in the left lateral position. Disappointingly, there was still a small percentage of midwives (5%) who had a strong preference for delivering women in the recumbent or lithotomy positions. Paradoxically, the most experienced midwives chose the recumbent position as their highest preference, while the least experienced midwives preferred the upright position.

Five core themes were identified with regard to midwives' reasons for choosing one position over another. These were perceived comfort for the women, familiarity with the chosen position, ability to give women choice and control, physical advantage for the women and physical accessibility for the midwife. From these, a 'dichotomy jigsaw' was constructed, in which midwives who had a strong preference for recumbent positions identified the importance of caring for their own physical health and having control over the women's body. This dichotomy has important implications for midwifery practice and is an important factor in the continuing trend to use recumbent and semi-recumbent positions today.

The findings also suggest that midwives are quite flexible in their approach, adapting and adopting different birthing positions even if they do not feel comfortable with the position or are inexperienced in its use, if requested to do so by the woman in their care. However, it is difficult to see how midwives who indicated such a strong preference for using the recumbent positions would, in reality, adjust their practice to suit the needs of the woman.

In addition, the majority of midwives (59%) regularly read the *RCM Midwives Journal*. By contrast, just under a third (27%) regularly read a second journal. There was also an association between those who read only one midwifery journal and a high preference for the use of recumbent positions. It may be that midwives who do not read widely may lack the evidence-based knowledge and impetus to change their practice, thus providing another reason for the use of recumbent positions in midwifery practice today.

Limitations of the study

This survey included the whole cohort of midwives (80) employed within a single midwifery unit with a delivery rate of just under 2000 per annum, and is therefore representative of the population of midwives within that unit. However, although the response rate was good, the total sample was small (n=66), therefore the results cannot be generalised to the whole midwifery population.

The survey was conducted at a time when the midwives were preoccupied with completing the caesarean audit, among other paperwork, and so the questionnaire may have been completed in haste. Moreover, some midwives may have conferred while completing the questionnaire, which could have further skewed the results. To minimise this effect, the researcher reminded the midwives to complete the questionnaire on their own, and provided a contact number should they have any queries.

Nevertheless, the findings are a significant step forward in understanding midwives' beliefs, attitude and preferences regarding the use of different birthing positions. The next logical step is to compare midwives' preferences for a particular birth position with those of the women in their care, to obtain further insight into current practice (see Chapter 9).

CHAPTER 7

Randomised controlled trial of focused *vs* general information in relation to birth position and decision-making

The systematic review described in the previous chapter highlighted gaps in the literature concerning choices, preferences and decision-making in relation to birth positions. It was evident that the methodology employed to address these issues was inappropriate in highlighting the needs and preferences of women in relation to their perception of choice and the decision-making process. It was hypothesised that the provision of focused information on the benefits of the upright birthing position would increase women's knowledge, decrease decisional conflict and help women decide which position to use for the delivery of their baby. The research methodology best suited to testing this hypothesis is a randomised controlled trial (RCT).

Randomised controlled trials

A RCT is a planned experiment designed to compare two or more forms of treatment or behaviour. The key factor in a controlled trial is the comparison of two groups that differ only with respect to their treatment (Altman, 1996). RCTs can be used to test the efficacy, effectiveness or equivalence of treatments and to test other healthcare practices and intervention strategies (Jadad, 1998; Peat, 2002). A meticulously designed and executed RCT is the gold standard of quantitative research (Gallo et al, 1995). It is the most commonly used experimental approach in the medical field; RCTs are sometimes referred to as 'true experiments' (Bick, 2000a). An RCT aims to demonstrate the presence or absence and magnitude of any causal relationship (Cluett, 2000; Cluett and Bluff, 2000). The study must be prospective because biases can occur when comparing groups treated at different times and possibly under different conditions (Altman, 1996). It should be comparative (controlled) and the absence of the treatment or intervention must also be taken into consideration. Biases cannot be ruled out if treatments are not randomly allocated (Bick, 2000a).

There are three main reasons why RCTs are considered the gold standard of research methods. First, the random allocation means that every participant has an equal chance of receiving the intervention. Second, the study groups tend to be similar with respect to all variables except for the intervention or treatment studied. Third, RCTs offer more conclusive evidence that the independent variable (in this case, focused information on the use of upright birthing positions) has an effect on the dependent variable (levels of knowledge and decisional conflict and confidence in decision-making). The delivery of the focused information was the intervention tested in this trial.

Strengths and limitations of experimental research

Few researchers would argue against the virtues of investing time and effort in an experimental study when testing the effects of an intervention or treatment. Indeed, true experiments are the most powerful method available to scientists for testing hypotheses of cause-and-effect relationships between variables (Sarantakos, 1998; Polit et al, 2001). Experimental research, especially a RCT, is also considered to provide the highest level of evidence for the effects of an intervention and for causation (Peat, 2002). A RCT is ideal for measuring short-term outcomes. However, large sample sizes are needed to measure significant differences, infrequent adverse outcomes or beneficial outcomes that are rare events. For example, a study to compare treatment intervention in women suffering from eclampsia with that in women with pre-eclampsia would require a large sample over time because eclampsia is a rare event.

Randomisation ensures that each subject has an equal chance of being allocated to a treatment or control group, and reduces the risks of inherent bias seen in other research designs. However, it is an unsuitable method for subjects with strong treatment preferences. For example, in a trial researching the efficacy of analgesia in labour, women with a strong preference for epidural analgesia would be reluctant to be assigned to the group without epidural analgesia. In addition, groups may not be comparable if subjects in the control group are reluctant or disappointed to receive the current treatment, and subjects in the experimental group are pleased to receive the new treatment. This can result in high drop-out rates or non-compliance during the experiment.

On the other hand, in experimental research, randomisation ensures that willingness to participate and other factors that may affect outcome do not influence group allocation. However, it may result in the exclusion of some patients to whom the results will subsequently be applied. For example, in midwifery research, ethical approval is only granted for clinical trials if women with a previous history of stillbirths are excluded, because of the need to protect such women from having to go through a choice of treatment. Yet, including cases such as these may highlight crucial factors in the quest to improve practice with regard to helping women with a previous history of stillbirth. Experimentation with human subjects is constrained by ethical considerations.

An experiment involves the creation of an artificial situation because the subjects, independent, dependent and extraneous variables and controls are precise and suggestive (Blaxter et al, 1996). Such artificiality has been criticised for not addressing the needs of subjects who wish to adapt or change their treatment.

Experimentation may not be feasible because it is impractical. For example, in the UK it is now impossible to study the effects of home and hospital births on outcome measures such as intervention rates, mortality or morbidity because the majority of women now deliver in hospital, making random allocation of women to home births or hospital births impractical. Selection bias would be an obvious problem. Also, any attempt to create an experimental condition between the home or hospital setting would be unrealistic because too large a sample or a multicentred trial would be required, rendering it unworkable.

Another limitation of experimental research is that a large number of human characteristics, such as sex, height, previous experiences and intelligence, cannot be experimentally controlled because they are not amenable to experimental manipulation (Polit and Hungler, 1983, 1999). It is not possible to randomly confer upon subjects a measurement of their intelligence, in order to observe the effect of their choice upon, say, home or hospital births. In some cases, the trial must be stopped if adverse effects are found in the treatment group; consequently, it will not continue for a sufficient period to measure long-term or adverse events. Conversely, if the results were overwhelmingly beneficial, then not to offer the treatment or intervention to all women would also be unethical (Cluett, 2000).

In addition, the views of subjects may change over time or be influenced by others (Sarantakos, 1998). If pre-testing is used, subjects may be sensitised and so be predisposed to the development of an interest in the experiment, leading them to respond atypically to experimentation. Historical events may occur between the pre-test and post-test, which may affect responses to the latter. For example, subjects may state that they do not know much about epidural analgesia. However, after watching a video of a woman having an epidural, the subject may decide strongly for or against its use, thereby introducing a confounding factor in the post-test analysis.

In addition, in experimental research, changes in the dependent variable may be due to changes in the pre-testing and post-testing rather than to the effects of the independent variable. This is known as measurement decay (Sarantakos, 1998). The Hawthorne effect, as discussed earlier, must also be taken into consideration, as the changes might be caused by the fact that the subjects know they are being studied. Finally, modelling effects must be taken into consideration: these occur when the dependent variable changes because the investigator expects the subjects to behave in a certain way or because subjects behave in a certain way to please the investigator (Sarantakos, 1998).

Although the major strength of experimental research is its ability to address causal relationships – invaluable in assessing the effects of different treatments or interventions – it is not error free, and can be time consuming, costly and discouraging. If the trial is not properly thought through, organised and thorough, evidence of bias, confounding variables and incomplete data could render it null and void.

The experimental process

In quantitative research, studies are conducted to determine the presence, type and degree of a causal relationship between two variables or treatment and the effectiveness of a specific intervention (Altman, 1996; Sarantakos, 1998; Clark, 2000). Experimental research involves five main processes:

1. Establishing and controlling the experimental conditions
2. Measuring the dependent variable
3. Introducing the independent variable
4. Testing the dependent variable
5. Assessing the presence and extent of change in the dependent variable (Sarantakos, 1998).

Various authors have described different approaches, with the number of stages or phases ranging from four to ten (Burns and Grove, 1993; Greenfield, 1996; Parahoo, 1997; Sarantakos, 1998; Polit and Hungler, 1999). Essentially, there are three key phases in planning an experimental research study. The first is the conceptual phase, i.e. the thinking, reasoning, planning and rationalising stage. This is an important phase, following which an appropriate research design and methodology is carefully selected. The next is the empirical phase. This can be both an exciting and laborious phase of the research. In this phase, data are collected by the researcher, interpreted and rigorously analysed to ensure that there are no accidental omissions or additions of data that could lead to inaccurate interpretation. Finally, there is the dissemination phase, when the results are presented, published and appraised by a wide audience. Research is pointless if this phase is forsaken, as it will mean that the opportunity to put the evidence into practice will be lost.

The strengths and qualities of experimental research make it the method of choice for determining the effects of an intervention to enhance women's ability to choose between the upright and recumbent position for childbirth.

Research hypothesis

The research study to be described here tested the hypothesis that the provision of focused information on the benefits of the upright position to pregnant women will significantly increase their knowledge, choice and use of upright birthing positions during labour.

Research question

In light of the hypothesis, the research question was: does focused information on the benefits of the upright position in labour influence women's choice and decision-making?

Aim

The aim of the study was to test the effectiveness of focused information on the use of birthing positions on women's decision-making process.

Objectives

° To provide a focused educational session on birth positions to pregnant women in preparation for childbirth
° To explore women's preferences for one type of delivery position over another.
° To introduce ADAPT (a decision analysis preference triage) as an instrument to help women make a decision on their choice of birthing position.
° To evaluate the value of focused information on collaborative decision-making between the woman and the midwife.

Methods

Research design

A double-blind randomised trial was conducted using a classic experimental or parallel design. The trial was 'double-blind' so that the intervention (focused information) was indistinguishable to both the women (participants) and the midwives who were caring for and assessing the women in labour. However, the nature of the trial meant that the researcher could not be 'blind' to the study throughout. To overcome the problems of researcher bias, a research assistant was recruited to assist in the random allocation of the women and to evaluate the delivery of information given by the researcher during the sessions. The role of the research assistant was to check the quality and quantity of the information given to the women in the experimental and control groups by the researcher.

Research setting

The main study was based in a maternity hospital in mid-Surrey with a delivery rate of approximately 2000 per annum and a full complement of 80 midwives, including bank midwives. During the study period (April 2000 to March 2001), the maternity unit had a normal delivery rate of 62%, an instrumental delivery rate of 13%, a caesarean rate of 24%, an induction rate of 18% and an augmentation rate of 38%.

Population and subjects

The unit from which the data were collected was located in an affluent area with a population of high caucasian origin. However, the study included pregnant women from all age and ethnic groups, parities and background, who were in the low-risk category. The reason for this was to ensure a diversity of interest during the random allocation process. All women in the last trimester of their pregnancy were invited to join the study.

Statistical issues

The power and probability of a study is an essential element in trials, ensuring that the results are not prone to type I or type II errors (Peat, 2002). Type I errors occur when a statistically significant difference is found, yet the magnitude of the difference is not clinically important, so that a finding of a difference between groups occurs when one does not exist. Type I errors usually arise when there is a sampling bias, or less commonly when the sample is very large or very small. Type II errors occur when a clinically important difference between two groups does not reach statistical significance; this happens when the sample is too small, or when researchers fail to find a difference between two groups when one truly exists (Peat, 2002). Erroneous rejection of the null hypothesis can occur in both type I and II errors (Polit and Hungler, 1999; Peat, 2002).

An adequate sample size is essential to ensure that there is a high chance of a clinically important difference between two groups reaching statistical significance. Advice on the total number of women required for the trial was taken from a reader in clinical and medical statistics. Using the appropriate statistical software, it was determined that the minimum number of women required to detect a difference significant at the 5% level with power 80% was 100 per group. A minimum of 200 women was therefore required for the trial. The power calculation for the determination of the group sizes was based on the expected rates of individuals, i.e. 65% and 45% for the experimental and control groups respectively, who will not change their initial decision on their choice of position during the second stage of labour The calculations were based on two confounding factors (variables) – parity and level of education – since both of these could affect the overall results if not taken into consideration. At every step of the trial, statistical advice was sought to ensure that the protocols were followed.

Sampling procedure

Women were randomly allocated to the experimental or control group by a stratified randomisation process, using a random grid, to ensure that each woman had an equal chance of being selected. An instrument (ADAPT) was developed as a decision aid to assist women in making their choices from eight different birthing positions more explicit by means of a scoring system (discussed in detail in Chapter 5). Women in both groups were then asked to evaluate to what extent their choice of birthing position or their decision to choose one position over another contributed to allaying decisional conflict and reducing decisional uncertainty.

A control group and an experimental group were established following responses to the letter of invitation. Because this was a double-blind trial, all participants were informed that they would be attending one of two sessions on 'Strategies for coping with labour', but neither the women nor the midwives caring for them would be aware of which group the women were allocated to. The purpose of double blinding is to reduce sampling and observer bias.

Stratified randomisation was used to keep the characteristics of the participants as similar as possible across the study groups (Jadad, 1998). To achieve this, two factors (or strata) known to be related to the outcome of the study were identified. These were parity and level of education. It was necessary to match for parity because women could have been influenced by previous labour and delivery experience. Level of education was considered symbiotic to level of social class. Studies have shown that women who attend classes are more educated and articulate, come from higher social classes and are more likely to attend parent education (Sturrock and Johnson, 1990; Mitchie et al, 1992; Lumley and Brown, 1993; Nichols, 1993; Nolan, 1995; Slade, 1996; Nolan, 1998). It was therefore important to match the participants evenly according to parity and level of education. A separate block randomisation scheme based on each factor was produced to ensure that the groups were balanced within each stratum.

Development and testing of the questionnaires

All the women in the trial completed a pre-test questionnaire (*Appendix 2*), two post-test questionnaires – the ADAPT decision instrument (*Appendix 1*) and a decisional conflict scale (*Appendix 3*) – and a post-delivery questionnaire to determine the birth outcome and level of collaboration between the midwife and the woman (*Appendix 4*).

In the context of this research study, a questionnaire is a set of standard questions administered to study participants for the purpose of gathering information or eliciting views for the study (Wagstaff, 2000). It has also been described as a structured self-report instrument, which may consist of a set of open or closed questions (Polit and Hungler, 1999; Polit and Beck, 2003). Questionnaires have the advantage over objective measurement tools, as they are simple and cheap to administer and can be used to collect information from the past or present (Peat, 2002). Questions within a questionnaire can be related to knowledge, behaviour, attitudes, opinions or beliefs (Sudman and Bradburn, 1982). To capture the interests of respondents, questionnaires should be well presented, readable and free from ambiguity. Thomas (1996) recommended that questionnaires should not be too long or complicated, and Oppenheim (1992) suggested that the phrasing should be limited to no more than 20 words per question. Pocock (1992) and Peat (2002) demonstrated that short questionnaires are more likely to achieve a better response rate than long questionnaires.

Treece and Treece (1986) recommend that a questionnaire should not be too tedious and take no more than 20–25 minutes to complete. On average, the midwives in the present survey study took about 12 minutes to complete the questionnaire, and the women about 14 minutes.

Reliability and validity

Reliability is the consistency with which a tool measures what it is intended to measure. Sudman and Bradburn (1982) identified four factors that may affect reliability or give rise to response error in surveys: memory, motivation, communication and knowledge. Memory is not always reliable, and if responders are not motivated or the study does not interest them it is unlikely that the questionnaire will be completed reliably. Poor communication about the purpose of the study may result in poor responses. Lack of knowledge about a particular subject or inability to understand the questionnaire may also affect reliability. One way to determine the reliability of a questionnaire is to put it through the test-retest process, in which individuals are asked to complete the questionnaire and then repeat it at a later date. Reliability is ensured when the responses to both questionnaires are similar (Polit and Hungler, 1999; Peat, 2002; Wagstaff, 2000).

Validity is an estimate of the accuracy of an instrument or the study results (Peat, 2002). It refers to the degree to which an instrument measures what it is supposed to measure (Polit and Hungler, 1999). There are two distinct types of validity. Internal validity is the extent to which the study methods are reliable and external validity is the extent to which the study results can be applied to a wider population.

Internal validity

A questionnaire or instrument has internal validity if its measurements and methods are accurate and repeatable. If a study has good internal validity then any differences in measurement between the study groups is attributed solely to the hypothesised effect under investigation (Peat, 2002). Internal validity of a questionnaire or instrument is situation specific because it applies only to similar subjects studied in a similar setting (Goodwin, 1997). Four main types of internal validity can be measured: face validity; content validity; criterion validity; and construct validity. Face validity will be discussed as it was applied to the research.

Face validity is sometimes called measurement validity. It is the extent to which an instrument measures what it is intended to measure and therefore tests the credibility of the instrument. Once a questionnaire has been peer reviewed, it must be tested on a small group of volunteers in a pilot study to ensure that it has good face validity. Good face validity is essential, as it is a measure of expert perception of the acceptance, appropriateness and precision of an instrument or questionnaire (Higgins, 1996; Polit and Hungler, 1999; Peat, 2002).

Each questionnaire was tested for face validity at the pilot stage and any ambiguity was amended in readiness for the trial. Reliability was assessed using the retest method described previously. All the questionnaires were given to the ethics committee for their comments. The questionnaires were developed as a prototype for the trial since this is the first study of its kind on birthing positions. However, elements of some of the questions were adapted from Mason (1989), who developed a survey to monitor the views of maternity service users.

ADAPT as a decision analysis instrument (revisited)

ADAPT is a decision analysis preference triage instrument. It measures degree of preference regarding women's choice of birthing positions on a five-point Likert scale. Women's explicit preference on the use of eight different birthing positions has never previously been evaluated in this way; this was the first time the instrument had been tested in a randomised trial. The only similar study was that of Dolan (1999), who developed a provider decision process assessment instrument to measure a healthcare provider's degree of comfort with a medical decision.

The ADAPT instrument was piloted on 20 women to test its validity. Ambiguity and problems in understanding the instrument were identified and corrected before it was used in the main study. Two minor changes were made. The pilot group felt that the the initial instructions were too long and wanted a brief overview, with verbal reinforcement from the researcher if required. Also, some women had difficulty in understanding the percentage rating (*Appendix 1*), stating that the 'neutral' rating was too high for them to make a definite decision, compared with the other ratings. For example, the 'neutral' stance on the ADAPT instrument was initially rated at 41–60%; this was considered too high, so the range was corrected to 40–59%, which was approved. This was then tested on five other women; no further problems were highlighted.

The instrument's test-retest reliability was tested using Pearson's correlation coefficient. This is a parametric test, which can be used to calculate data from ratio scales measurement. Repeatability is sometimes referred to as reproducibility, consistency, reliability, or test-retest variability. Repeatability is a measure of the consistency of a method and the extent to which an instrument produces the same result when used in the same subject on more than one occasion (Peat, 2002). The test-retest reliability based on the sample of 20 women was significant at the $P<0.01$ level for all eight positions, confirming the validity and reliability of ADAPT as a useful instrument for decision-making.

All participants were asked to complete a questionnaire before and after the educational input (intervention) to evaluate the effect of the intervention.

Application of a decisional conflict scale

A decisional conflict scale (DCS) (*Appendix 3*), adapted from that of O'Connor et al (1999), was used to evaluate the ADAPT instrument. O'Connor (1995) developed a DCS in response to the lack of instruments available to evaluate healthcare consumer decision aids. The DCS is used to tailor decision-supporting interventions to consumer needs. In the present study, the DCS was used to measure the women's attitude towards the use of the various birthing positions, and to evaluate the extent of their decisional 'conflict' concerning their certainty and uncertainty about the choices made. The test-retest reliability coefficient of the DCS developed by O'Connor was 0.81, based on a sub-sample of 909 individuals (O'Connor, 1995). This means that the DCS discriminated significantly (P<0.0002) between those who had strong preferences for a particular birthing position and those who were uncertain about their decisions.

Women completed the DCS using a five-point Likert scale. This is one of the most common scales used to measure attitudes, being simple and easy to complete and requiring respondents to select their attitude to a particular statement from a small number of ordered alternatives (Wagstaff, 2000).

Post-delivery questionnaire for participants and midwives

To increase validity, both the study participants and the midwives were 'blind' to the study. One of the main outcomes of the study was the extent of collaboration between the mother and the midwife, based on their known or unknown preferences. To measure this outcome, at the end of the delivery the midwives were asked to complete a short questionnaire (*Appendix 6*) to identify the final delivery position and the extent of collaborative decision-making, and provide details of the birth for the data analysis.

Levels of measurement

A combination of nominal and ordinal levels of measurement was used in the questionnaires. For example, nominal measurement was used when women were asked about their parity and level of education. Ordinal measurement was used for data classified into discrete categories, such as when women were asked to identify how important it was for them to be able to use their highest scoring birthing position, based on four categories – very important, important, not so important and not important at all.

Ratio measurement was used in the ADAPT decision instrument when women were asked to rate their preferences for each of eight birthing positions on a scale of 0–100%. Ratio measurement allows for a score of zero to be analysed as an absolute value (Smart, 1997). Interestingly, when Pearson's correlation analysis was performed, based on 212 women who completed the ADAPT questionnaire correctly, an inverse relationship was found, in that women who gave a high rating to the semi-recumbent position also tended to give as high a score to all the other conventional positions, such as lateral, recumbent and lithotomy; conversely, those who gave a high score to an upright birthing position, such as kneeling, tended to score all the other upright positions similarly. This correlation was significant at $P<0.01$.

Ethical considerations

During the past two decades in the UK, every study involving human participants has had to to obtain ethics committee approval before the research can proceed, to ensure that vulnerable subjects are not included and that the treatment or intervention is safe and ethically appropriate.

For this particular study, the researcher (author) held several meetings with the midwifery managers, staff and obstetricians at an early planning stage to assess the feasibility of conducting the research and involving the mothers and the staff. A plan to conduct an observation study in the delivery suite to evaluate how midwives cope with care and delivery of a mother in relation to choice of birthing positions, in the presence and absence of a delivery bed, was proposed.

However, after two meetings with staff in 1997, this idea was abandoned because it was felt that some of the staff, and indeed some mothers, would not be able to cope with delivering a baby in the absence of the bed. Similarly, it was apparent that some staff would feel threatened by the presence of an observer during this crucial stage of labour. In addition, it was intimated that the researcher was expected to be on-call for 24 hours of the day for the proposal to work with the staff. Obviously, this was neither practical nor realistic. The observation proposal was therefore abandoned. However, feedback concerning a research study on birthing positions was positive, and several midwives at the meeting provided encouragement, highlighting a need for research on birthing positions.

In the spring of 1998, two further meetings were held between the midwifery managers, obstetricians and staff, concerning the feasibility of conducting a RCT comparing the effects of focused information on birthing positions *vs* general information on strategies for coping with labour. This proposal received a positive response, and a full research composite was therefore submitted to the appropriate district medical ethics committee in December 1999. The proposal included a background to the study of birthing positions, aims and objectives of the study, details of the target population, and an introduction to the new measurement scale (ADAPT, *Appendix 1*) developed by the researcher to identify women's choice and decision with reference to eight birthing positions. Information about the right of participants to accept, refuse or withdraw from the study was also highlighted.

Before the study, participants signed the consent form, which included additional information, such as the role of the researcher and the participants, details of data collection and confidentiality. The form also contained details of the pilot study, which explained how participants would be selected. The researcher met with the ethics committee panel to discuss the proposal and clarify any queries. Approval was obtained in March 2000, following some modifications: for example, the researcher should provide a statistician with an account of the study to check statistical viability, and should give midwives the opportunity to attend an educational session on the use of various positions in labour to allay any anxiety in those midwives who were unfamiliar with the use of upright postures.

The conditions were noted and all the midwives were invited to attend an educational session on birthing positions. Following the pilot study, some minor modification to the educational plan was required, e.g the information on birthing positions was more detailed for the experimental group than the control group, and the educational session was increased from 60 minutes to 90 minutes to give women in both groups more time to complete the questionnaire and the new 'decision' instrument developed by the researcher.

The intervention

The intervention consisted of delivery of the 'focused information' to the experimental group, and a 'placebo' session (general information about strategies for coping with labour) to the control group. The intervention was conducted by the researcher, supported by the research assistant, who helped with scribing and technical details during each session. Each session lasted approximately 90 minutes. The experimental groups were given evidence-based information on the use of different birthing positions. A variety of educational methods were used in the delivery of the information. For example, an overheard projector was used to show illustrations of the positions, and the researcher demonstrated how women could adopt each position. The experimental group were also shown a 15-minute video of a woman delivering in the standing position. The control group watched a video on 'exercises in pregnancy' and were given a session on the use of different forms of pain relief in labour.

Structure of the focused and general information

To ensure that the delivery of the information to the experimental and control groups by the researcher was consistent from one session to the next, the researcher followed an itemised checklist of issues to be discussed at each session (*Appendixes* 7 and 8). The research assistant then assessed this list at each session to provide an objective evaluation. Any comments made by the assistant were taken into consideration in preparation for the next session.

Overall, there was very little deviation from the list. Of the 20 sessions provided to each group, only two deviated slightly from the original: in one session, to the experimental group, information on nutrition and hydration in labour was inadvertently omitted; and in another session, to the control group, information on using water for relaxation was left out. Neither omission affected the overall outcome.

Outcome measures

There were four main outcome measures for this study:

1. The level or degree of knowledge on birthing positions before and after the intervention
2. Women's preferences for eight different birthing positions
3. Level of decisional conflict in the decision-making process
4. Uptake of the upright position in labour and childbirth in relation to women's choice and decision-making process.

Response rate

A final sample of 517 women for the main study and 176 for the pilot were entered into the study. A total of 369 women from the main study replied within 2 weeks, giving an overall response rate of 71%. Of these, 259 (70%) were eligible for entry to the main study. However, 24 women did not arrive for the session. The remaining 235 women were entered into the main trial, including 20 women who were initially invited to participate in the pilot group, but were not selected for it. Thirteen women were transferred out to deliver in another area. A further eight women had their baby before receiving the letter of invitation. Twelve women replied that they were going to have a caesarean. Sixty-nine women were willing to answer any questionnaires in support of the study, but did not wish to attend the session. Various reasons were given: they could not find the time to attend (22); they had attended a parent education session (18) or were too busy with other children (9); six women had to work till the end of the pregnancy and three did not feel well enough to travel. Eleven women did not give any reasons. Data collection was completed by mid-January 2001.

Data collection approaches

Once full ethics approval had been obtained for the trial, the researcher met with the delivery suite manager, midwives and community midwives to explain the details of the study and the extent of their involvement. The researcher was given permission to obtain participants' details from the database in the IT unit, following a session on how to access the computers within the unit for the purpose of the research. Initially, at the suggestion of the midwives, the plan was to involve the community midwives so that they could distribute the information and invitation to participate in the study. A designated room in the researcher's home was identified as the place to store all the information and data from the participants, ensuring confidentiality and safekeeping of research data. These were kept in four coloured-coded boxes and files and labelled according to the month of delivery.

There were two phases to the trial. In the first phase, women whose babies were due in April 2000 were invited to participate in the pilot study. In the second phase, women whose babies were due in August, October and November 2000 were identified through the hospital computerised data system. These months were chosen so that the study would not coincide with the National Caesarean Audit in May and June and the Baby Friendly Breastfeeding Audit in August. As the educational sessions were held approximately 4 weeks before delivery, the month of August did not clash with the Baby Friendly Audit. Each month the hospital database generated a list of 150–175 women who were expected to give birth during August, October and November 2000.

A letter was sent to all the women explaining the nature of the study, and their consent to participation in the trial was obtained. They were invited to attend a 90-minute session on 'Strategies for coping with labour'.

Data were collected from eligible women in the antenatal period from the 32nd to the 40th week of gestation. The potential suitability of women in the last trimester of their pregnancy had been discussed with the manager and staff in the unit. The last trimester was considered the most appropriate as most working women would be on maternity leave and feel more able to take time off to attend the session. Also, general parent education sessions are available during this time for all antenatal women. This approach therefore ensured consistency of data collection.

A total of 118 women in the experimental group were randomly allocated to the focused session, where they were given information on the evidence for and against the use of different positions in labour. A total of 117 women in the control group were given a general (placebo) session on 'strategies for coping with labour', which concentrated mainly on the use of pain relief in labour.

Inclusion criteria

° Pregnant, regardless of parity, due for delivery in August, October or November 2000.
° Willing to participate.
° Ability to understand the English language.

Exclusion criteria

° Booked for elective caesarean section.
° Booked for water-birth.
° Booked for elective epidural analgesia
° Do not understand or speak English.
° Do not wish to participate, for whatever reason.

Before embarking on the main research, a pilot study was conducted with 20 women. Of these, 12 were randomly allocated to the control group and eight to the experimental group. The questionnaires were tested on this sample and any ambiguities found were resolved before the start of the main trial.

Figure 7.1 shows a flow chart of the total number of women entered into the pilot study and the main trial.

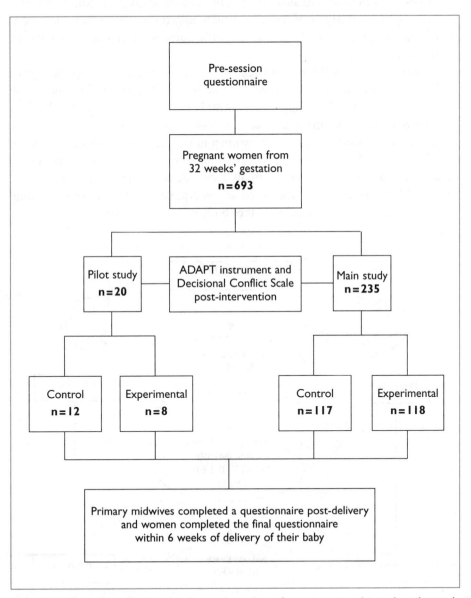

Figure 7.1: Flow chart showing the the total number of women entered into the pilot study and the main trial.

Data analysis

All the entries from the questionnaires were tabulated, coded and itemised individually by the researcher, and cross-checked by the statistician. Data were analysed using SPSS 10.0 statistical software package and Microsoft Excel databases from February to June 2001. Chi-squared analysis, a non-parametric test, was used for analysis of the data. Where appropriate, significant and non-significant differences will be shown, with degrees of freedom (df) where appropriate.

Figure 7.2 depicts the model used by the researcher to develop the trio of studies. The three studies are interrelated and interwoven in that they show how the results of the RCT are applicable to midwives. The results of the RCT in Chapter 8 highlight to the midwifery profession what women want and how midwives can support and empower women in their decision-making. Chapter 9 describe the midwives' survey, which highlights the dichotomy that exists between midwives' knowledge of midwifery care and what occurs in practice. Chapter 10 concludes with a discussion and interpretation of the results, detailing how this research has contributed to the 'body of midwifery knowledge'.

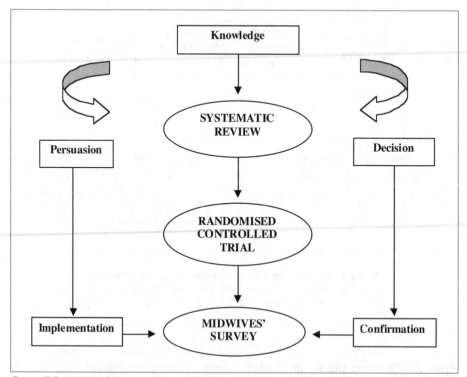

Figure 7.2: Model of three studies within Roger's theoretical framework.

CHAPTER 8

Results of the randomised controlled trial

The results of the randomised controlled trial (RCT) of the effects of focused information *vs* general information in relation to birth position and decision-making are presented in this chapter and Chapter 9. A total of 235 women participated in the trial, of whom 117 were randomised to a control group (general information) and 118 to an experimental group (focused information). The results are presented in five categories: demographic and baseline data; ADAPT instrument analysis; decisional conflict scale (DCS) analysis; mothers' post-delivery responses; and midwives' post-delivery responses. The first three categories of results are presented here and the last two categories in Chapter 9. Discussion of the findings and the conclusion follow in Chapter 10.

Demographic and baseline data

The educational level and age of the women in the experimental and control groups are summarised in *Figure 8.1*. The women were asked to identify their highest educational attainment; the results were then grouped into three levels: level 1 (GCE/GCSE); level 2 (A level/diploma); level 3 (degree/masters or higher).

Figure 8.1 shows that the two groups were similar with respect to age, both having a peak in the age group 26–35 years. Level of education was also evenly distributed across the groups, except for a slight increase in level 3 in the

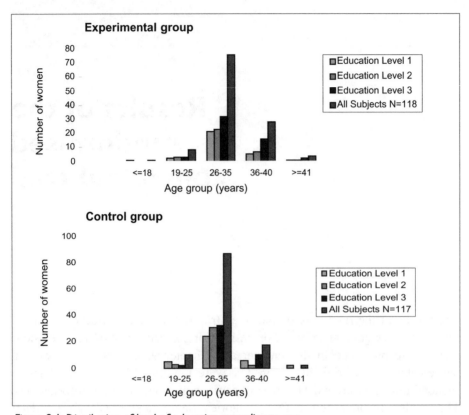

Figure 8.1: Distribution of level of education according to age.

experimental group for the age group 36–40 years (16 experimental *vs* 10 control), and in level 2 in the control group for the age group 26–35 years (31 control *vs* 24 experimental). However, none of these differences were significant (chi-squared = 5.4, P=0.8 [experimental] and chi-squared = 12.6, P=0.2 [control], 8df).

Randomisation was achieved using stratified random sampling, with parity and level of education as the variables to ensure a similar distribution in the two groups. The findings would not therefore be expected to show any differences in these variables between the groups, and this was the case (*Figure 8.2*).

In addition, age and parity were found to be evenly distributed across the educational levels, with no significant differences between the groups (chi-squared = 1.295, P=0.6, 2df). The two groups entered into the trial were therefore well matched for parity and level of education, hence the true effect of the independent variable on the dependent variables could be measured.

Attendance at parent education before the intervention in the experimental and control groups was comparable. However, fewer women in the experimental group had attended parent education compared with the control

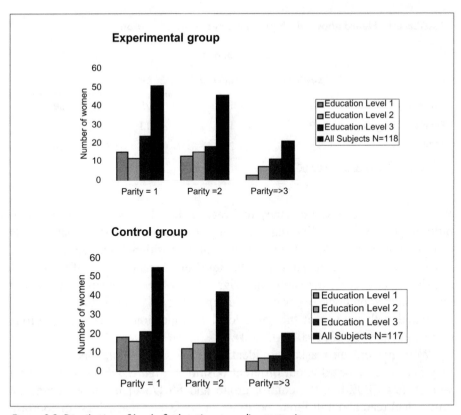

Figure 8.2: Distribution of level of education according to parity.

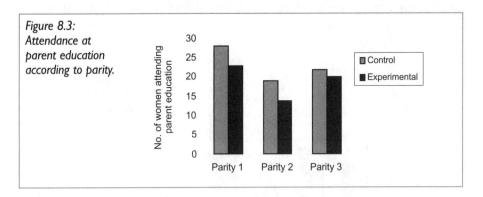

group, but the differences were not significant (chi-squared = 0.202, P =0.95; 2df). Sixty-nine (59%) women in the control group and 57 (48%) in the experimental group had attended parent education classes, giving an average of 54% who had attended parent education held by the midwives. *Figure 8.3* shows a breakdown of the number of women who attended parent education, according to parity.

TABLE 8.1: Heard about birth positions in parent education

	Educational level			Total
	Level 1	*Level 2*	*Level 3*	
Control group	13	12	25	50
Experimental group	9	12	13	34
TOTAL	22	24	38	84

Chi-squared = 16.323, P<0.0001, 2df

Women were asked whether they had read or heard about different types of birthing positions for delivering their baby. The findings showed that only 84 (36%) women had read or heard about birthing positions in parent education. The data were then matched against the level of education to see if there were any differences. *Table 8.1* shows that significantly fewer women at the highest level of education in the experimental group had heard about birthing positions, compared with women at the same level of education in the control group (chi-squared = 16.323, P<0.0001, 2df).

Women were also asked to identify, from six possible options, where they had read or heard about different positions. *Figure 8.4* shows that most women (94 ([80%] in the control group and 86 [73%] in the experimental group) had read about different positions in books and magazines. In contrast, only 50 (43%) women in the control group and even fewer (34; 29%) in the experimental group had obtained their information from parent education.

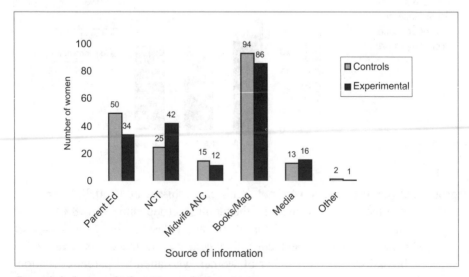

Figure 8.4: Source of information on birth positions.

Knowledge rating before the intervention

Women were asked to rate their knowledge of different birthing positions on a scale of 1–10. The majority of scores were in the range 3–8, indicating that most women had more than a little knowledge to a lot of knowledge. *Table 8.2* shows that most women had an average score, at scale point 5-6. There were no significant differences between the groups at any point on the scale; this ensures homogeneity within the groups before the intervention, which in turn reduces the problems of sampling error (Jadad, 1998; Polit and Hungler, 1999; Peat, 2002; Polit and Beck, 2003).

TABLE 8.2: Knowledge of birthing positions before the intervention

			Scores			
	0–2	**3–4**	**5–6**	**7–8**	**9–10**	**Total**
Control group	9	28	58	18	4	117
Experimental group	2	30	70	13	3	118
TOTAL	*11*	*58*	*128*	*31*	*7*	*235*

Chi-squared = 1.108, P=0.9, 4df   Not significant

Before the intervention, all the women were asked whether, in the last trimester of their pregnancy, they had thought about a particular position in which they would like to deliver their baby. The responses from the groups were evenly distributed: in the control group 50% had thought about positions and 50% had not thought about it, and in the experimental group 49% had thought about positions and 51% had not thought about it.

Those women who had thought about a particular position were then asked if they could specify which position they would like to adopt for the delivery of their baby. They were asked to specify three positions from a list of eight. For statistical analysis, the eight positions were grouped into two categories: recumbent (which included recumbent, semi-recumbent and lateral) and upright (standing, squatting, semi-squatting, all fours and kneeling). In both the control and experimental groups, more women specified a decision to use the upright position for childbirth than specified the recumbent position, although the difference was not significant. The responses are summarised in *Table 8.3*. The total numbers reflect the multiple responses given by the women.

Even when the choices were extrapolated to the top five popular choice of positions, where semi-recumbent position was identified as the most common choice by both groups of women, no significant differences were found (*Table 8.4*).

TABLE 8.3: Choice from two categories of birthing position

	Recumbent*	Upright†	Total
Control group	67	92	159
Experimental group	58	106	164
TOTAL	*125*	*198*	*323*

Chi-squared = 1.288, P=0.8, 1df   Not significant

*Recumbent includes recumbent, semi-recumbent and left lateral positions

†Upright includes standing, squatting, semi-squatting, all-fours and kneeling positions

---

TABLE 8.4: Choice of five birthing positions before the intervention

	Semi-recumbent	Squatting	Semi-squatting	All-fours	Kneeling
Control group	45	11	21	24	26
Experimental group	44	24	21	35	19
TOTAL	*89*	*35*	*42*	*59*	*45*

Chi-squared = 1.542, P=0.9, 4df   Not significant

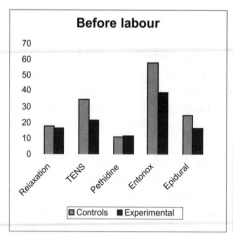

Figure 8.5: Choice of pain relief before labour.

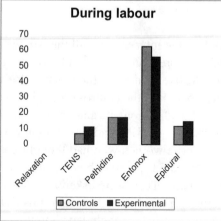

Figure 8.6: Choice of pain relief during labour.

Women were also asked to specify their choice of pain relief before labour. In both groups, more women thought that they would like to try entonox, with pethidine being the least favoured form of pain relief. Differences in the choice of pain relief between the groups were not significant (chi-squared = 0.777, P=0.95, 4df; *Figure 8.5*).

When compared with actual pain relief used, the results were very similar, although *significantly* more women in both groups used entonox for pain relief than used the other forms of pain relief. Interestingly, fewer women in the control group than the experimental group actually used epidural analgesia in labour. Conversely, fewer women in the experimental group actually used TENS compared with their pre-labour decision, although the differences were not significant in either group (chi-squared = 0.191, P=0.99, 3df; *Figure 8.6*).

The midwives did not perceive relaxation techniques to be a form of pain relief and therefore comparisons could not be made.

ADAPT – an instrument for analysing decision preferences

Following the intervention, all the women were asked to complete ADAPT, a 12-item questionnaire developed as a decision instrument to help women decide which birthing positions to use during labour (*Appendix 1*). They could also choose not to complete the questionnaire. Consequently, two women from the control group and one from the experimental group did not complete the questionnaire as they were in a hurry to leave the session. A further seven women in the control group and one in the experimental group either completed the questionnaire incorrectly or did not fully complete it. In total, there were 108 completed questionnaires from the control group and 116 from the experimental group for analysis.

Both groups were asked to rate their knowledge of birthing positions on a scale of 1–10. The data were analysed by combining the ratings into three categories: nil to little knowledge (scores 0–3); some knowledge (scores 4–6); a lot of knowledge (scores 7–10). A comparison of knowledge levels before and after the intervention for the experimental and control groups is shown in *Table 8.6*. Significant differences before and after the intervention were found in both groups; however, the difference was highly significant in the experimental group (P<0.0000001) compared with the control group (P<0.0001).

Table 8.5 also shows a 13-fold increase in knowledge levels rated 4–6 in the experimental group after intervention, compared with just over a twofold increase in the control group.

Significant differences were also found when the knowledge levels between the control and experimental groups post-intervention were compared (*Table 8.6*). The same data are presented in *Figure 8.7*.

Figure 8.7 illustrates the differences in knowledge score ratings between the control and experimental groups. Although both groups gained knowledge after the intervention, the experimental group gained *significantly* more

TABLE 8.5: Knowledge levels before and after the intervention

	Nil to little (0–3)	Some (4-6)	A lot (7–10)	Total
Control group				
Pre-session	24	66	20	110
Post-session	43	0	74	108
TOTAL	67	66	94	218

Chi-squared = 58.794, P<0.0001, 2df

	Nil to little (0–3)	Some (4-6)	A lot (7–10)	Total
Experimental group				
Pre-session	22	79	16	117
Post-session	0	6	110	116
TOTAL	22	85	126	233

Chi-squared = 1154.820, P<0.0000001, 2df

TABLE 8.6: Comparison of knowledge levels post-intervention

	Nil to little (score 0–3)	Some (score 4-6)	A lot (score 7–10)	Total
Control group	4	30	74	108
Experimental group	0	6	110	116
TOTAL	4	36	184	224

Chi-squared = 26.792, P<0.000001, 2df

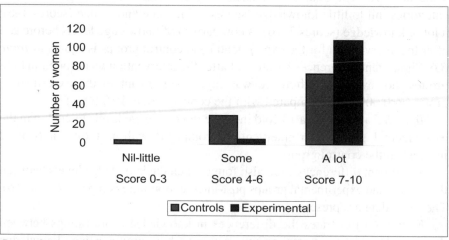

Figure 8.7: Comparison of knowledge ratings for control and experimental groups post-intervention.

knowledge following the focused information session. Moreover, none of the women in the experimental group rated their level of knowledge of birth positions below 5 post-intervention.

Women were then asked to rate their preferences for eight different birthing positions: the recumbent, semi-recumbent, left lateral, kneeling, squatting, semi-squatting, standing and all-fours positions. The preference scores were combined into three categories for analysis: very weak to weak preference (0–39%); neutral or no preference (40–59%); strong to very strong preference (60–100%). *Table 8.7* compares the preferences for the experimental and control groups for all the upright positions. Highly significant differences between the control and experimental groups were found for all the upright positions, the only exception being the all-fours position, where the difference was not significant (P=0.4).

The preference results for all birth positions were then combined into two categories: recumbent (lying flat on the bed, semi-recumbent, and left lateral) positions and upright (squatting, semi-squatting, all fours, standing and kneeling) positions. Results for the control and experimental groups are compared in *Figure 8.8*.

TABLE 8.7: Choice of upright birth position

	Very weak to weak	*Neutral or no preference*	*Strong to very strong*
Squatting			
Control group	44	28	32
Experimental group	28	21	67
	Chi-squared = 16.323, P<0.0001, 2df		
Semi-squatting			
Control group	38	20	47
Experimental group	13	13	90
	Chi-squared = 26.755, P<0.00001, 2df		
Standing			
Control group	38	28	38
Experimental group	18	35	63
	Chi-squared = 3.494, P<0.005, 2df		
Kneeling			
Control group	24	17	65
Experimental group	10	12	94
	Chi-squared = 1.489, P<0.005, 2df		
All fours			
Control group	24	17	64
Experimental group	20	14	82
	Chi-squared = 2.331, P=0.4, 2df Not significant		

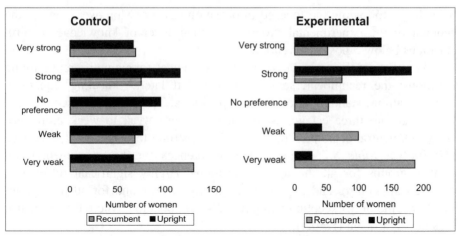

Figure 8.8: Birth position preferences when combined into two categories: recumbent and upright.

In the control group, preferences for the recumbent position *vs* upright position were not significantly different (chi-squared = 7.025, P=0.20, 4df). In contrast, preferences for the upright *vs* recumbent position in the experimental group revealed a *highly significant* difference (chi-squared = 62.860, P<0.00001, 4df; *Figure 8.8*). The results also showed an inverse relationship in that between the weak and very strong preferences, the experimental group was very strongly in favour of upright positions, whereas the control group was less in favour of upright positions but more strongly in favour of recumbent postures; conversely, more women in the control group than the experimental group had a very weak preference for upright postures.

All the women were asked to give their reasons for the position they rated least preferable. The three main reasons cited are summarised in *Table 8.8*. These were: first, it was the least comfortable; second, the women were influenced by the research studies discussed during the session; and third, it appeared the least natural. Significantly more women in the experimental group than in the control group were influenced by the research studies discussed during the session. This difference was significant at P<0.05.

TABLE 8.8: Three main reasons for choice of least preferred position

	Least comfortable	*Research studies*	*Least natural*
Control group	58	31	54
Experimental group	68	71	67
TOTAL	126	102	121
Chi-squared = 6.723, P<0.05, 2df			

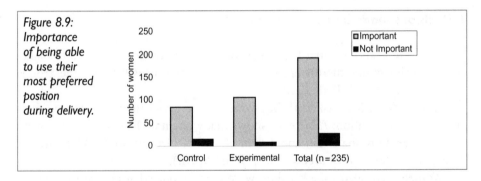

Figure 8.9: Importance of being able to use their most preferred position during delivery.

Women were also asked how important it was for them to be able to use the position they rated their highest preference for delivery. *Figure 8.9* shows that more women in the experimental group considered it to be very important or important to be able to use their most preferred position, which, in this case, was the ability to adopt the upright posture. However, the difference between the two groups was not significant (chi-squared = 3.448, P=0.1, 1df).

Decisional conflict scale analysis

It was important to evaluate ADAPT as a decision aid in order to establish its value in quantifying uncertainty and the factors contributing to uncertainty, both during the process of deliberation and after the choices had been made. Following completion of the ADAPT instrument, the women in the study were asked to complete the DCS to measure the extent of their certainty or uncertainty while making their choices of birthing positions and pain relief during labour.

Responses to the DCS were divided into four categories:

1. Decisions made under uncertainty
2. Factors contributing to uncertainty
3. Perceived effective decision-making with reference to birth positions
4. Perceived effective decision-making with reference to pain relief.

Eight questionnaires from the control group and one from the experimental group were incomplete and were omitted from the analysis, which was therefore based on 100 completed questionnaires from the control group and 116 from the experimental group. As the differences in sample size were small, the sample was considered appropriate for analysis (Bailey J, 2001, personal communication).

1. Decisions made under uncertainty

Women were asked whether their decision on birth position was hard to make. *Table 8.9* shows that there were no significant differences between the groups (chi-squared = 5.304, P=0.1, 2df).

Women were then asked if they were unsure about their decision on their choice of birth position. *Table 8.10* shows that women in the control group were *significantly* more uncertain about their choice of birth position (47 control *vs* 74 experimental; chi-squared = 7.252, P<0.05, 2df).

Women were also asked if they were clear about what choice of position was best for them. *Table 8.11* shows that *significantly* more women in the experimental group agreed or strongly agreed that they were clear which choice of position was best for them (41 control *vs* 67 experimental; chi-squared = 6.098, P<0.05, 2df).

TABLE 8.9: 'Decision on birth position hard to make'

	Agree or strongly agree	Neither agree nor disagree	Disagree or strongly disagree	Total
Control group	36	20	44	100
Experimental group	40	12	64	116
TOTAL	*76*	*32*	*108*	*216*

Chi-squared = 5.304, P=0.1, 2df   Not significant

TABLE 8.10: 'I'm unsure what to do'

	Agree or strongly agree	Neither agree nor disagree	Disagree or strongly disagree	Total
Control group	22	31	47	100
Experimental group	22	20	74	116
TOTAL	*44*	*51*	*121*	*216*

Chi-squared = 7.252, P<0.05, 2df

TABLE 8.11: 'Clear what choice is best'

	Agree or strongly agree	Neither agree nor disagree	Disagree or strongly disagree	Total
Control group	41	33	26	100
Experimental group	67	24	25	116
TOTAL	*108*	*57*	*51*	*216*

Chi-squared = 6.098, P<0.05, 2df

2. Factors contributing to uncertainty

In the second section of the DCS, women were asked whether they were aware of the choices on different positions in labour, in order to ascertain factors contributing to uncertainty. *Table 8.12* shows that both groups were aware of the different choices on positions in labour, but the differences between the groups were not significant.

Following the educational session, both groups were asked if they needed more information about choices on birth positions. *Table 8.13* shows that *significantly* more women in the control group than in the experimental group felt that they needed more information (chi-squared = 8.967, $P<0.025$, 2df*)*.

All the women were asked if they knew about the benefits of using upright positions for delivery. *Table 8.14* shows that *significantly* more women in the experimental group knew about this (chi-squared = 9.918, $P<0.01$, 2df).

TABLE 8.12: 'Aware of choices on different positions in labour'

	Agree or strongly agree	Neither agree nor disagree	Disagree or strongly disagree	Total
Control group	36	20	44	100
Experimental group	40	12	64	116
TOTAL	76	32	108	216

Chi-squared = 5.304, P=0.1, 2df   Not significant

TABLE 8.13: 'I need more information about choices on birth positions'

	Agree or strongly agree	Neither agree nor disagree	Disagree or strongly disagree	Total
Control group	12	29	59	100
Experimental group	6	20	90	116
TOTAL	18	49	149	216

Chi-squared = 8.967, P<0.025, 2df

TABLE 8.14: 'Knowledge of the benefits of upright positions for delivery'

	Agree or strongly agree	Neither agree nor disagree	Disagree or strongly disagree	Total
Control group	90	7	3	100
Experimental group	115	0	1	116
TOTAL	205	7	4	216

Chi-squared = 9.918, P<0.01, 2df

TABLE 8.15: 'I feel it is too soon for me to make a decision on choice of birth positions'

	Agree or strongly agree	Neither agree nor disagree	Disagree or strongly disagree	Total
Control group	32	18	50	100
Experimental group	20	15	81	116
TOTAL	*52*	*33*	*131*	*216*

Chi-squared = 9.243, P<0.01, 2df

TABLE 8.16: 'I am pleased to be given the choice to make a decision before I go into labour'

	Agree or strongly agree	Neither agree nor disagree	Disagree or strongly disagree	Total
Control group	81	15	4	100
Experimental group	109	6	1	116
TOTAL	*190*	*21*	*5*	*216*

Chi-squared = 8.646, P<0.025, 2df

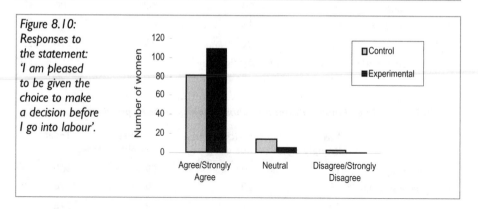

Figure 8.10: Responses to the statement: 'I am pleased to be given the choice to make a decision before I go into labour'.

All the women were in their last trimester (median 37.2 weeks) when they attended the educational session. They were asked if it was too soon for them to make a decision on their choice of birth positions. *Table 8.15* shows that *significantly* more women in the experimental group than in the control group disagreed that it was too soon for them to make a decision on birth positions (chi-squared = 9.243, P<0.01 2df).

Once they had made their decision, both groups were asked if they were pleased to be given a choice to make their decision on birth positions before going into labour. *Table 8.16* and *Figure 8.10* show that more women from both groups agreed or strongly agreed that they were pleased to be given a choice. However, *significantly* more women in the experimental group were pleased to

TABLE 8.17: '*It would help to be reminded of the benefits of the upright position*'

	Agree or strongly agree	Neither agree nor disagree	Disagree or strongly disagree	Total
Control group	72	16	12	100
Experimental group	95	11	10	116
TOTAL	*167*	*27*	*22*	*216*

Chi-squared = 3.107, P=0.3, 2df   Not significant

TABLE 8.18: '*Hard to decide if the benefits of upright positions are more important than the benefits of conventional delivery*'

	Agree or strongly agree	Neither agree nor disagree	Disagree or strongly disagree	Total
Control group	23	24	53	100
Experimental group	6	16	94	116
TOTAL	*29*	*40*	*147*	*216*

Chi-squared = 21.447, P<0.00001, 2df

be given a choice to make a decision before they went into labour (81 control *vs* 109 experimental; chi-squared = 8.646, P<0.025, 2df).

Women were asked if it would help to be reminded about the benefits of the upright position when they go into labour. *Table 8.17* shows that most women thought it would help to be reminded of the benefits of using the upright position, but there were no significant differences between the groups (72 control *vs* 95 experimental; chi-squared = 3.107, P=0.3, 2df).

Women were asked if they found it hard to decide whether the benefits of upright positions were more important to them than the benefits to be gained from using the conventional delivery position. This question served to clarify women's understanding of the benefits of upright positions compared with recumbent positions. Only one woman (from the control group) did not answer this question. *Table 8.18* shows that *significantly* more women in the control group, compared with the experimental group, were uncertain about the benefits of using the upright position (23 control *vs* 6 experimental; chi-squared = 21.447, P<0.00001, 2df; *Table 8.19*).

3. Perceived effective decision-making with reference to birth positions

Perception of the effectiveness of the decision made on birth position was ascertained in the third section of this scale. Women were asked if they felt that they had made an informed choice on their decision regarding birth positions. *Table 8.19* shows that there was a *highly significant* difference between the control group and the experimental group. Although *significantly* more women in the experimental group felt that they had made an informed choice regarding their preferences for birth positions, compared with the control group (35 control *vs* 15 experimental; chi-squared = 12.343, P<0.005, 2df), the majority of women from both groups were non-committal in their responses (59 control *vs* 70 experimental).

Women were asked if they expected to stick with their decision on choice of birth position when they were in labour. Significantly more women in the experimental group than the control group agreed or strongly agreed that they would stick to their decision when they were in labour (63 experimental *vs* 30 control; chi-squared = 13.298, P<0.005, 2df; *Table 8.20* and *Figure 8.11*).

TABLE 8.19: 'I feel I have made an informed choice'

	Agree or strongly agree	Neither agree nor disagree	Disagree or strongly disagree	Total
Control group	15	59	26	100
Experimental group	35	70	11	116
TOTAL	*50*	*129*	*36*	*216*

Chi-squared = 12.343, P<0.005, 2df

TABLE 8.20: 'I expect to stick with my decision'

	Agree or strongly agree	Neither agree nor disagree	Disagree or strongly disagree	Total
Control group	30	58	12	100
Experimental group	63	46	7	116
TOTAL	*93*	*104*	*19*	*216*

Chi-squared = 13.298, P<0.005, 2df

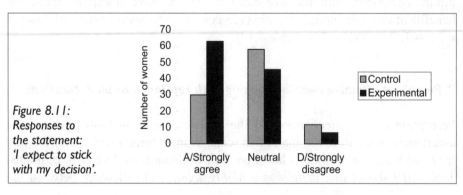

Figure 8.11: Responses to the statement: 'I expect to stick with my decision'.

TABLE 8.21: 'Decision I made was the best decision possible for me'

	Agree or strongly agree	Neither agree nor disagree	Disagree or strongly disagree	Total
Control group	8	56	36	100
Experimental group	17	78	21	116
TOTAL	25	134	57	216

Chi-squared = 9.843, P<0.01, 2df

Irrespective of whether or not the decision that the women made on birth positions was personally the best decision possible for them, *significantly* more women in the experimental group felt that their decision to use the upright position was the best decision for them (chi-squared = 9.843, P<0.01; *Table 8.21*).

4. Perceived effective decision-making with reference to pain relief

Perceived effectiveness of the decision made on pain relief was ascertained in the last section of this scale, where women were asked if they expected to stick with their decision on their choice of pain relief. *Table 8.22* shows that a *highly significant* number of women in the experimental group expected to stick with their decision compared with women in the control group (chi-squared = 11.012, P<0.005, 2df).

TABLE 8.22: 'I expect to stick with my decision [with reference to pain relief]'

	Agree or strongly agree	Neither agree nor disagree	Disagree or strongly disagree	Don't know	Total
Control group	41	50	7	2	100
Experimental group	70	32	9	5	116
TOTAL	111	82	16	7	216

Chi-squared = 11.012, P<0.005, 2df

Finally, no significant differences between the experimental and control groups were found in relation to whether women felt that they had made an informed choice regarding their choice of pain relief, and whether they were satisfied that the decision they had made on pain relief was consistent with their personal values. Satisfaction with, and importance of, decision choice regarding pain relief in the experimental and control groups was also similar.

CHAPTER 9

Mothers' and midwives' post-delivery responses

Mothers' post-delivery responses

Birth outcomes and decision-making

All the women in the trial were asked to complete a single questionnaire (*Appendix 2*) after they had delivered their baby, to enable evaluation and comparison of the effectiveness of focused and general information on decision-making during labour. The questionnaire contained 13 questions in total; the last question invited the women to add any further comments on their decision-making in labour. All comments were categorised to identify common themes. These will be described at the end of this section.

Most women returned the questionnaire within 6 weeks. Sixty-six (28%) reminders were sent out within a month of delivery. Of these, 29 (44%) were returned completed within 2 weeks. Overall there was a good response rate, with 106 (91%) women from the control group and 114 (97%) from the experimental group returning the questionnaire. This level of response was high compared with other studies; Coppen (1984), for example, achieved a 67% response rate in a survey of women's views of maternity care. The face-to-face contact that the women had with the researcher may have motivated the women to reply. Also, a stamped addressed envelope was enclosed with the questionnaire, which was printed on coloured paper as this has been found to yield a better response rate in previous studies (Eastwood, 1940).

Table 9.1 shows that 70 women in the control group and 71 women in the experimental group had a normal delivery. The majority of the women delivered

TABLE 9.1: 'Did you have a normal delivery?'

	Yes	No	No reply	Total
Control group	70 (60%)	36 (31%)	11 (9%)	117 (100%)
Experimental group	71 (60%)	43 (36%)	4 (3%)	118 (100%)
TOTAL	141	79	15	235

Chi-squared = 3.890, P=0.2, 2df Not significant

in the hospital. Nine mothers (5 from the experimental group and 4 from the control group) delivered at home; all of these adopted the upright position. However, for consistency and homogeneity, only the responses from the women who had a normal delivery and delivered in the hospital were analysed.

To evaluate the effectiveness of focused information/education on collaborative decision-making between the woman and the midwife, it was important to determine to what extent the educational session facilitated collaboration with the midwife during labour. Interestingly, *significantly* more women in the experimental group than the control group were able to collaborate with their midwife (chi-squared = 14.539, P<0.001, 2df, *Figure 9.1*).

Women had been asked to identify their choice of delivery position following the intervention, so it was important to see whether women were able to collaborate with the midwife who looked after them during labour on their decision about which position to use for delivery. *Table 9.2* shows that more

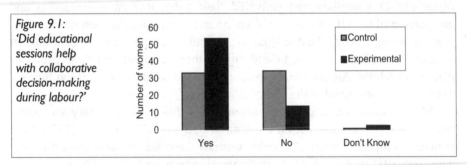

Figure 9.1: 'Did educational sessions help with collaborative decision-making during labour?'

TABLE 9.2: Ability to collaborate with midwife on decision about delivery position

	Yes, and used predetermined position	Yes, collaborated but did not end up with my choice	No	Total
Control group	24	15	31	70
Experimental group	31	19	21	71
TOTAL	55	34	52	141

Chi-squared = 3.278, P=0.2, 2df   Not significant

TABLE 9.3: Value of educational session on decision-making during the first stage of labour

	Unhelpful or helped a little	Moderately helpful	Helped a lot or very helpful	Total
Control group	12	24	34	70
Experimental group	3	21	47	71
TOTAL	15	45	81	141

Chi-squared = 7.680, P<0.025, 2df

TABLE 9.4: Value of educational session on the ability to focus on choice during the second stage of labour

	Unhelpful or helped a little	Moderately helpful	Helped a lot or very helpful	Total
Control group	8	33	29	70
Experimental group	10	23	38	71
TOTAL	18	56	67	141

chi-squared = 3.210, P=0.3, 2df   Not significant

women in the experimental group were able to use their predetermined choice of upright positions and were able to collaborate more easily with their midwife on their decision, but the differences were not significant.

Table 9.3 shows that *significantly* more women in the experimental group than the control group found the educational session on women's decision-making process in the first stage of labour of value (chi-squared = 7.680, P<0.025, 2df). However, when the women were asked whether the educational session helped them to focus on their choice of position during the second stage of labour, there were no significant differences between the groups (P=0.3). Nevertheless, more women in the experimental group than the control group found that the educational session helped a lot or was very helpful (*Table 9.4*).

Women were asked whether they preferred any particular birth position during the course of labour or whether they were indifferent. *Figure 9.2* shows that although the majority of the women from both groups (62 control and 55 experimental) had a preference for a particular birth position, only 52% (32) of the control group and 44% (24) of the experimental group actually delivered in their preferred position, but the difference between the groups was not significant (chi-squared = 0.168, P=0.95, 2df).

When asked if they would have liked more time to make a decision about which position to use for delivery while they were in labour, a small group of women (28; 19%) felt they needed more time to make a decision, but most

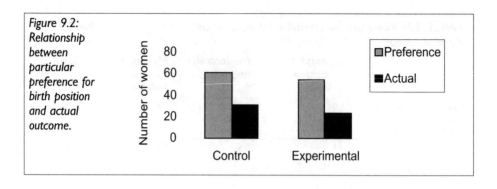

Figure 9.2: Relationship between particular preference for birth position and actual outcome.

TABLE 9.5: Would you have liked more time to make a decision on the position to use in labour?

	Yes	No	Don't know	Total
Control group	11	55	4	70
Experimental group	17	51	3	71
TOTAL	28	106	7	141

Chi-squared = 1.573, P=0.5, 2df   Not significant

women (106; 74%) felt that that they did not need more time. There were no significant differences between the groups (*Table 9.5*).

Interestingly, although half the women did not deliver in their position of choice, the majority were very satisfied with their decision on birth position. However, eight women from the experimental group were dissatisfied with the outcome of the birth position. All these women chose the upright position, but were refused: six because of the need to monitor, consequently they had to lie on the bed; one was too tired to stand; and another was told by the midwife that she could not deliver in the upright position. No significant differences were found between the experimental and control groups (*Table 9.6*).

When asked whether the educational session helped them to make an informed decision about other issues in pregnancy or labour, more women in

TABLE 9.6: Satisfaction with decision made on birth position

	Dissatisfied	Satisfied	Very satisfied	Total
Control group	5	20	45	70
Experimental group	8	12	51	71
TOTAL	13	32	96	141

Chi-squared = 3.060, P=0.3, 2df   Not significant

TABLE 9.7: Did the educational session help you to make an informed decision about other issues in pregnancy or labour?

	Yes	No	Don't know	Total
Control group	58	11	1	70
Experimental group	66	4	1	71
TOTAL	124	15	2	141

Chi-square = 3.776, P=0.2, 2df   Not significant

TABLE 9.8: How important is it to be fully informed about any decision to be made while in labour?

	Very important	Important	Quite important	Not important at all	Total
Control group	58	11	0	1	70
Experimental group	62	9	0	0	71
TOTAL	120	20	0	1	141

Chi-squared = 1.326, P=0.6, 2df   Not significant

the experimental group (66) compared with the control group (58) responded positively, although the difference was not significant (*Table 9.7*).

Women were asked how important it is to be fully informed about any decision that is to be made while in labour. As expected, most women in both groups felt it was very important or important to be fully informed, and the difference was not significant (*Table 9.8*).

Qualitative analysis of women's decision-making process

Women were asked if they wanted to make any further comments about the decision-making process that they experienced while in labour. *Significantly* more women in the experimental group (53; 75%) made one or more comments compared with women in the control group (24; 34%) (chi-squared 6.199, P<0.025, 1df). Three themes emerged from analysis of these comments:

- The value of the educational session
- The difficulties in making decisions during labour
- The impact of the unpredictability of labour on decision-making.

A selection of the comments are reproduced below to illustrate how these themes emerged. Care has been taken to include the views of women from both groups.

The following comments are from women who received educational input in the experimental group. They highlight the value of the educational session in:

- increasing their knowledge
- increasing their confidence
- increasing their awareness of the options available
- being in control.

> *'The session I attended was excellent...'*
>
> *'Your session gave me knowledge, which gave me confidence so I wasn't scared during labour or delivery. It was a great help.'*
>
> *'The session was definitely helpful as my first labour was traumatic and problems arose postnatally. Before the session I had not made up my mind about choosing between elective caesarean or normal delivery. I am glad I chose the latter.'*
>
> *'After the session I felt more confident in choosing positions and collaborating with the midwife in early labour...'*
>
> *'Your advice on using the birthing ball was very good for the length of labour and I was able to try all the positions you recommended to get comfortable.'*
>
> *'I found seeing you very very helpful because going on all fours in labour helped me enormously.'*
>
> *'The session was extremely useful as I was able to be more assertive with the midwife, although she was extremely helpful anyway.'*
>
> *'I was incredibly pleased to have a normal delivery, being 34, a doctor, IVF pregnancy, but the session gave me added confidence; I was more mobile and laboured at home most of the time.'*

The second theme to emerge was the difficulties that women experienced in decision-making and collaborating with their midwife during labour. Three factors were expressed within this theme:

- being monitored
- communication barrier between the midwife or doctor
- not being able to predict events in advance.

Comments expressing these factors included:

> *'Due to being strapped to the monitor for the last hour of the first stage, I couldn't be in the position I wanted, which was the standing position, and this was very frustrating...'*

'During the first stage, I think I could have discussed positions for delivery more fully, but once in bed, there was no discussion...doctors rushed in, legs were in stirrups...'

'When pushing, midwife thought semi-reclining with stirrups to open the pelvis would assist as my baby was in the occipito-posterior position [lying with head facing upwards, rather than face down (occipito-anterior) in the normal position], but I wanted to squat!'

'The first midwife I had did not make me feel very comfortable and did not discuss the various options...'

'Decisions and options need to be made and considered before labour as time is needed to communicate to the midwife the options, and the midwife needs to respect individual wishes.'

'It was nice to discuss with the midwife but when they changed shifts it seemed that they hadn't communicated, for example, husband cutting the cord, position preferences...'

'Care received from midwives varied. First midwife said she would use a Sonicaid to listen to the baby, thus allowing me to be in any position. Then shift changes, and new midwife was adamant that I was to be monitored!'

The third theme that emerged concerned the impact of the unpredictability of labour on decision-making. Comments expressing this theme included:

'Sometimes the situation calls for immediate assistance and no time is left for decision-making.'

'Any personal decision or preference cannot really be 100% decided in advance as it is necessary to go with the flow of the particular labour.'

'I delivered 1 hour 45 minutes after arrival at the delivery suite so there was not much time to use any positions for labour.'

'I think it is very important to be well informed. However, it is also important not to be too unrealistic as things don't always go according to plan and you may have to change'.

'I would probably try something different, that is, more upright positions next time round, as I am more aware of what labour is really like!'

'I would have liked to have tried other upright positions, but being monitored and the speed of delivery didn't enable me to do so.'

Overall, therefore, women were very pleased with the information they received from the educational session. However, *significantly* more women in the experimental group than the control group commented on the value of being fully informed about adopting upright positions during labour and childbirth (chi-squared = 61.99, P<0.025, 1df).

Midwives' post-delivery responses

The midwives who were responsible for the delivery of the women were asked to complete a single-sheet questionnaire following delivery of the baby. Two months into the start of the main trial, however, it became clear that many midwives were not completing the questionnaire. A brief meeting with some of them followed to try to resolve the problem. Reasons given by the midwives for non-completion included feeling that they were already having to complete so many documents soon after delivery, such as the birth notification, the main birth record book kept in the delivery suite, and the client's case notes, that there was no time for any more. Also, having completed a lengthy questionnaire for an earlier caesarean audit, the midwives in the delivery suite felt that it was tedious to have to complete yet another questionnaire. In addition, the researcher felt that perhaps the novelty of the research, which began with a pilot study in April, had waned, and perhaps the midwives were unable to appreciate the importance of their contribution to the research.

To ease the process, the researcher and her assistant agreed to complete the section of the questionnaire requiring factual information that was easily accessed, such as date of birth, parity, name of mother and type of delivery. The midwife completed the section that required her professional judgment, such as whether the mother adopted different positions in labour and the method of pushing. This made it possible for the questionnaire to be completed more readily by the midwives. However, two questionnaires from the control group and one from the experimental group were missing, and were therefore excluded from the analysis.

There was a fairly even distribution of women who delivered between 37 and 40 weeks' gestation and those who delivered at term in both groups (*Table 9.9*).

Parity of the women was well matched between the control and experimental groups (*Table 9.10*). There were slightly more multiparas than primiparas in both groups, but the difference between the groups was not significant.

The mode of delivery was identified by the midwives and double-checked via birth records for accuracy. These were grouped into normal, forceps

---

TABLE 9.9: Comparison of groups by weeks of gestation

	<37 weeks	37–40 weeks	>40 weeks	Total
Control group	4	55	56	115
Experimental group	0	51	66	117
TOTAL	4	106	122	232

Chi-squared = 4.954, P=0.1, 2df   Not significant

TABLE 9.10: Parity of the women

	Primiparas	Multiparas	Total
Control group	52	63	115
Experimental group	51	66	117
TOTAL	103	129	232

Chi-squared = 0.014, P=0.95, 1df   Not significant

TABLE 9.11: Mode of delivery

	Normal	Instrumental	Caesarean	Total
Control group	79 (67%)	19 (16%)	19 (16%)	117
Experimental group	76 (64%)	13 (11%)	29 (24%)	118
TOTAL	155	32	48	235

Chi-squared = 3.262, P=0.2, 2df   Not significant

Figure 9.3: Mode of delivery.

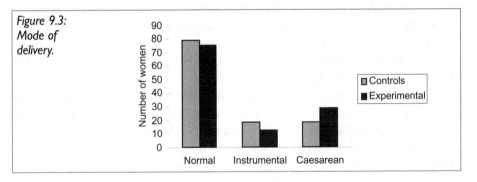

(including ventouse) and caesarean. The mode of delivery for both groups in terms of normal and forceps delivery rate were very similar; more women had a caesarean in the experimental group, but the differences were not significant (*Table 9.11* and *Figure 9.3*).

The average length of labour was 6 hours 10 minutes in the experimental group and 7 hours 7 minutes in the control group. The longest labour for a mother having her first baby was 19 hours 9 minutes and the shortest labour for a mother having her third baby was 1 hour 10 minutes in the experimental group and 21 hours 59 minutes and 1 hour 39 minutes respectively in the control group. There were no significant differences in the length of labour for all three stages in both groups (P=0.7). However, women in the experimental group generally had a shorter labour as a whole. Overall, midwives' highest preference for a particular position was associated with the actual position used to deliver the women. However, the numbers for each stage of labour were too small to make any accurate comparisons between the groups.

TABLE 9.12: Positions attempted during the second stage of labour

	Control group	Experimental group	Total
Recumbent	1	0	1
Semi-recumbent	49	54	103
Left lateral	15	18	33
Lithotomy	2	3	5
Semi-squatting	5	4	9
Squatting	1	1	2
Standing	10	13	23
All fours (hands and knees)	18	16	34
Kneeling	18	34	52
Dorsal	0	1	1
TOTAL	*119*	*144*	*263*

Ten different positions were attempted during the second stage of labour (*Table 9.12*). The five most common positions were the semi-recumbent, left lateral, all fours, standing and kneeling positions. The semi-recumbent position still featured high on the agenda of positions used by the midwives in both groups. However, significantly, almost twice as many women in the experimental group used the kneeling position during the second stage, compared with the control group (34 experimental *vs* 18 control). The totals reflect the multiple positions that women adopted during the second stage, and show that more women in the experimental group attempted more than one position compared with the control group, although the differences were not significant.

TABLE 9.13: Actual position adopted for delivery

	Control group	Experimental group	Total
Recumbent (flat in bed)	4	3	7
Semi-recumbent	44	40	84
Left lateral	10	7	17
Lithotomy	0	1	1
Semi-squatting	0	2	2
Squatting	1	1	2
Standing	1	2	3
All fours (hands and knees)	2	2	4
Kneeling	7	13	20
Dorsal	1	0	1
TOTAL	*70*	*71*	*141*

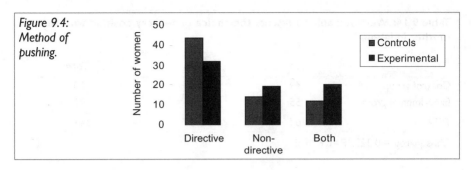

Figure 9.4:
Method of
pushing.

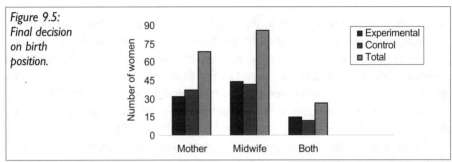

Figure 9.5:
Final decision
on birth
position.

The actual position used to deliver the baby did not show any significant differences between the groups (*Table 9.13*). However, twice as many women adopted the kneeling position in the experimental group compared with the control group (13 experimental *vs* 7 control).

Midwives were asked to identify the method of pushing used at the second stage of labour, from a choice of directive, non-directive or both types. Most midwives used directive or active pushing: 44 (63%) in the control group *vs* 32 (45%) in the experimental group. A smaller group of midwives used indirect or passive pushing: 14 (20%) in the control group *vs* 19 (27%) in the experimental group. However, there were no significant differences between the groups (chi-squared = 4.645, P=0.1; 2df; *Figure 9.4*).

It was important to determine who made the final decision on the choice of delivery position as this would indicate the extent to which women were empowered to make their own choice during this crucial stage of labour. The responses show that, in the control group, midwives made the final decision 42% of the time and mothers made the decision 37% of the time. Similar rates were found in the experimental group, where midwives made the decision 44% of the time and mothers made the decision 32% of the time. Ranking third is the joint decision made between the mother and the midwife (12 in the control group and 16 in the experimental group). The obstetrician also featured in this decision, although only two women had the decision made by the doctor. However, the differences were not significant in any of the groups (P=0.1). *Figure 9.5* summarises the data for the three highest groups.

Table 9.14: Were you able to discuss the choice of delivery position with the mother in labour?

	Yes	*No*	*Total*
Control group	49	21	70
Experimental group	55	16	71
TOTAL	*104*	*37*	*141*

Chi-squared = 0.325, P=0.6, 1df

Although more midwives made the final decision on the choice of delivery position, most of them were able to discuss the option with the mother. Nevertheless it was surprising that the midwife did not discuss the choice of position with amost a third (21; 30%) of the women in the control group and a quarter (16; 23%) of the women in the experimental group (*Table 9.14*).

There was no significant difference in blood loss following delivery between the groups: median blood loss was 235 ml (control) *vs* 225 ml (experimental).

More women in the experimental group received a second-degree tear. However, the same group sustained fewer episiotomies than the control group, but there were no significant differences between the groups (chi-squared = 0.098, P=0.995, 4df; *Figure 9.6*).

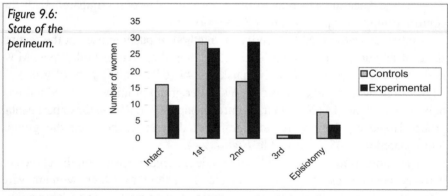

Figure 9.6: State of the perineum.

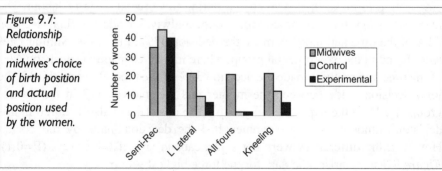

Figure 9.7: Relationship between midwives' choice of birth position and actual position used by the women.

Finally, the midwifes' strongest preference for a particular birth position was matched against the actual position used by the women during the second stage of labour. *Figure 9.7* shows that there was an association between midwives' preference for the semi-recumbent position and the actual position used during the second stage (*Figure 9.7*). In contrast, the all-fours position featured least in both the control and experimental groups.

CHAPTER 10

Discussion of the findings and conclusion

A total of 235 women took part in the trial: 117 were randomly allocated to the control group and 118 to the experimental group. Women from both groups were well matched for age, parity and level of education, although women in the experimental group were slightly more educated at level 3 but the difference between the groups was not significant.

Studies have shown that women who participate in research are often better educated and from a higher social class (Nichols and Humerick, 1988; Mason, 1989; Slade and MacPherson, 1993; Brown and Lumley, 1998; Hanson, 1998a). Social class was not identified in this study because it is well documented that social class based on partner's occupation is not a good indicator of a woman's attitude (Graham, 1984; McFarlane and Mugford, 1984; Oakley, 1986). Educational level is a better predictor of women's attitudes (Husband, 1983; Green et al, 1990; Browner et al, 1996). Also, women's educational attainment at the time of booking has been shown to be a better predictor of attendance at parent education classes than social class. Parity was identified as it was thought that women's previous experiences may affect their knowledge and choice of birthing positions. Parity and level of education were therefore two possible confounding variables.

How useful are parent education classes?

An average of 54% of women in the trial had attended parent education classes and there was no significant difference between the experimental and control groups. In contrast, Michie et al (1992) found that as many as 81% of women in their study had attended at least one parent education class. It may be that some women in the current trial have yet to attend parent education, as they entered the trial in their last trimester, a time when most women would begin antenatal classes. This may account for the differences. On the other hand, Nolan (1995) pointed out, in her small study, that there may be duplication of attendance at antenatal classes. She found that 23% of 78 first-time couples attending hospital classes, 61% of 36 first-time mothers attending National Childbirth Trust (NCT) classes and 48% of 25 women attending Active Birth classes were also going to a second set of antenatal classes. Understandably, she called for a rationalisation of services.

Attendance at antenatal classes has generally never been high, and only half of all expectant parents attend classes (Amos et al, 1988; Jacoby, 1988; Murphy-Black, 1990; Coppen, 1994). Nolan (1995) found that women from social classes 4 and 5 and the very young were almost entirely unrepresented, yet these groups of women are at greater risk of developing problems in pregnancy and therefore have a greater need of parent education than others.

Some women, however, choose not to attend parent education because they do not find it useful, as identified by the researcher during the current trial. One mother in her second pregnancy said: *'I did not find it useful the last time.'* Another said: *'They keep talking about pain in labour, but I wanted to know more about coping with the pain'*. In contrast, some women in the trial thought that previous attendance precluded them from attending again – *'I have already attended parent education'* was a common comment. A mother having her second baby said: *'I was not invited this time round'*. The poignant remark from another mother, who said *'just because this is my third baby does not mean that I do not want to attend classes'*, highlights the assumption that midwives had made regarding her need for more information.

Clearly, the findings concur with previous studies (Boyd and Sellars, 1982; McCabe et al, 1984; McIntosh, 1988), which cited similar reasons for poor attendance at antenatal education by women, e.g. the classes were not worthwhile, attended classes in a previous pregnancy, and women's lack of awareness of the classes. The findings indicate that midwives should not assume that parent education is only for first-time mothers; antenatal education needs to be pertinent and useful enough to meet the needs of all mothers if it is to be of any value (Murphy-Black, 1990; Slade, 1996).

Only one third (36%) of the women in the trial had heard about birthing positions in parent education classes, and fewer women in the experimental group at educational levels 1 and 3 (9 and 13 respectively) had heard about birthing positions, compared with the control group (13 and 25 respectively). However, the differences were not significant. This meant that two-thirds of women in the trial had not heard about birthing positions during parent education classes. Women cannot be expected to know what is best for them or make an informed decision if they are unaware of the numerous options available. Yet successive government reports have emphasised the importance of informing women and making them aware of the available options so that they can make an informed choice (Maternity Services Advisory Committee, 1982, 1984, 1985; House of Commons Health Select Committee (Winterton Report), 1992; Department of Health, 1993; National Institute for Clinical Excellence (NICE), 2003; Wanless Report, 2004; Department of Health, 2004, 2005). I could not agree more with the recent recommendation from the NICE (2003) that *'addressing women's choices should be recognised as being integral to the decision-making process'*.

Over the past decade, much time and effort has been spent on highlighting the need to provide sufficient and unbiased information to women so that they can make an informed decision. For example, a government-supported initiative to produce evidence-based, informed choice leaflets for dissemination to women was launched in 1996 (NHS Centre for Reviews and Dissemination, 1996). The leaflets were written in lay terms so that they were easy to understand. The information in the leaflets was based on research evidence. Women were informed about the different choices available to them with regard to birthing positions. The midwife's role was to disseminate the information and provide women with a choice of options without bias, so that the women could make an informed decision. However, the extent to which midwives have used the leaflets to inform women is largely unknown.

The findings in this study show that only one-third of women in the trial had been informed about birthing positions in parent education classes. Yet parent education is an ideal time for midwives to provide evidence-based information to women; armed with such information and the informed choice leaflets, women should be well prepared by the time they go into labour. Unfortunately, studies have shown that women may not translate what they have learnt in parent education classes into practice (Copstick et al, 1985; Niven 1986; Green, 1993; Slade et al, 1993). In their study of women's expectations and experiences, Slade et al (1993) found that women expected to be able to use their coping strategies more, and have more control over their pain, than they actually did while in labour. Copstick and colleagues (1985) argued that professionals could no longer assume that women who have been taught coping techniques in labour would necessarily be able to use them. In a large survey of women before and after labour, Green (1993) found that 79% of women wanted to use breathing and relaxation exercises during labour. However, only 63% actually used these exercises all or most of the time, 27% used them for a while and 10% did not use them at all. It was concluded that an association between antenatal class attendance and use of strategies existed only for relaxation methods (Niven, 1986; Slade, 1996).

When women in the current trial were asked where they had heard about different birthing positions, surprisingly the majority of the control group (94; 80%) and the experimental group (86; 73%) identified books and magazines as the source of their information. A much smaller number of women in the control group (50; 43%) and even fewer in the experimental group (34; 29%) had heard about positions from parent education classes. Most women, therefore, were not as well informed about birthing positions from parent education classes as they were from reading books and magazines. More women in the experimental group (42; 36%) than the control group (25; 21%) had heard about birthing positions from NCT classes. This may be because less than half the women in the experimental group had heard about positions during parent education classes, and therefore felt the need to attend NCT classes.

Yet it is argued that if women are to have real choice, two prerequisites are necessary, namely information and research (Mander, 1993). There is no doubt that demand for a higher standard of care, choice and control for women has led to information and research becoming both a reality and a necessity (Department of Health, 1993; Clinical Standards Advisory Group, 1995; Audit Commission, 1998; NICE, 2003; Wanless Report, 2004). The need to provide women with real choice through the delivery of information and research-based evidence has never been more urgent than now. Parent education is one method whereby midwives can deliver information and empower women to increase their knowledge of important issues that are relevant to their needs (Robertson, 1994).

Before the intervention, women were asked to rate their knowledge of different positions on a scale of 1–10 to establish that there were no significant differences and to exclude any prior influences on their knowledge level from obtaining information about birthing positions from other sources. Results showed no significant difference in the knowledge scores between the groups, with most women obtaining an average knowledge score of 5.

It was also important to determine whether women had any prior thoughts about a particular position in which they would like to deliver their baby. The findings in the two groups were strikingly similar, with an almost equal number of women in each group having thought about a particular position they would like to adopt for delivery before the intervention. When the findings were grouped into those who wished to use a recumbent position and those who wished to use an upright position, it was found that more women wanted to use an upright position, but there were no significant differences between the groups. In contrast, of those who were able to identify the types of positions they would like to use to deliver their baby, the majority wanted to use the semi-recumbent position rather than any of the upright positions.

Women identified the semi-recumbent position as their ideal choice, with the left lateral and fully recumbent positions as second and third choices, respectively; only a fifth of the women had thought about delivering in the semi-squatting, all-fours or kneeling position. Sleep (1990) suggested that this may reflect 'Hobson's choice', for unless women undergo preparatory exercise and education programmes during pregnancy, endorsed by positive encouragement to try alternative positions during labour, they are unlikely to feel sufficiently confident to follow their own inclinations – highlighting once again the need for informed choice.

Many studies on antenatal education have focused on the need to provide adequate information by challenging the teaching and the educator to provide information that meets women's needs (Robertson, 1994; Rees, 1996; Nolan, 1998). Other studies have discussed the role of antenatal education in reducing anxiety about a particular issue in first-time mothers (Hibbard et al, 1979; Libbus and Sable, 1991; Hoddinott and Pill, 1999) or focused on the benefits of an educational programme as a whole (Redman et al, 1991; Murphy-Black, 1990; Slade, 1996). Many of these studies were descriptive and discussed the basis of antenatal education in broad terms; they did not compare different educational strategies or demonstrate how positive encouragement to use the upright position can be provided to women in labour.

The lack of information on birthing positions at parent education classes was highlighted by the finding that only 36% of women had heard about birthing positions from this source, with the majority of women (80%) obtaining their information on birthing positions from books and magazines. These results highlight gaps in current antenatal education and demonstrate the need to provide women with more information on positions in labour. Indeed, the benefits of focused information and education on women's knowledge of birth positions, and their ability to choose one type of position over another with confidence, have not been tested before.

Choice, preferences and knowledge of birthing positions

The ADAPT decision instrument was developed to ascertain the degree and extent of women's preference for one type of position over another. First, it asked women to rate their knowledge of birthing positions before and after the intervention in order to determine the effectiveness of the focused information in increasing level of knowledge. No significant differences were found in the level of knowledge before the intervention between the control and experimental groups (P=0.5). Following the intervention, however, both groups had a significantly increased level of knowledge, and significance was almost three times stronger in the experimental group (P<0.0000001) than in the control group (P<0.001).

These findings confirm that focused information is effective in increasing knowledge levels. Interestingly, they also show that women in the control group might have experienced a degree of 'Hawthorne effect' during the trial, in that their knowledge of birthing positions increased significantly despite not being given any focused information on birthing positions. It may be that more women in the control group were already well informed about birthing positions through previous experiences and/or books, and the minimal information given to them on birthing position was sufficient to increase their knowledge of it.

Although the researcher tried to ensure consistent delivery of information to both groups throughout the trial, some women from the control group may have received more information on birthing positions than the researcher intended. This could have occurred during the opening session when women were invited to ask questions. If a question on birthing positions arose, the researcher felt obliged to give that information to the whole group as it would have been unethical to withhold such information from other participants. This may explain the significant differences in knowledge level found in the control group pre- and post-intervention. Nevertheless, the evidence clearly shows that the provision of focused information on birthing positions significantly increased the level of knowledge of women in the experimental group. It therefore enables rejection of the first null hypothesis (that the provison of focused information on the benefits of the upright birthing position will not have any effect on the level of knowledge), as a significant difference between the effects of focused information and general information on women's level of knowledge was found in this study.

The findings concur with those of Hillier and Slade (1989), who assessed women's knowledge levels before and after a course of antenatal classes. They found significant increases in knowledge after the classes. However, women in Hillier and Slade's study were self-selected and there was no control group.

Women in the current trial were then asked to rate their preferences for eight different birthing positions. Analysis of the findings showed that women in the experimental group were consistently giving almost all the upright positions significantly higher preference ratings compared with women in the control group. The exception was the all-fours position, which both groups of women rated a very strong preference. The findings therefore demonstrate that focused information on the evidence for and against the use of different birthing positions had a significant effect on the preferences of women in the experimental group.

In addition, when the results were grouped into two distinct categories, i.e. recumbent and upright positions, significant differences were found between the groups. The experimental group indicated a significantly greater preference for upright positions than recumbent positions ($P<0.0001$), whereas the control group was neutral, and differences between their preferences for recumbent and upright positions were not significant ($P=0.1$). The demonstration of significant differences in women's preferences for one type of position over another when focused information was provided allows rejection of the second null hypothesis (that the provision of focused information on the benefits of the upright position will not have any effect on woman's choice or preferences for upright positions).

The evidence also shows that significantly more women in the experimental group were influenced by the research studies discussed during the session on birthing positions ($P<0.05$), thereby attesting to the value of providing evidence-based information to women to help them decide which birthing position to use (NICE, 2003; Wanless Report, 2004). The results also provide evidence that women's choice of birthing position can be influenced by research studies. Walsh (1998) obtained similar results in a study of midwives: after attending a course on the use of upright positions, 46% of midwives in the study were using upright positions in their practice compared with 11% before the course.

Following the completion of ADAPT, a decision aid to help women decide which birthing position to use, all the women in the trial were asked to complete a decisional conflict scale (DCS) to enable quantification of any decision uncertainty while making their choice of birthing position. The results provide an indication of both the value of ADAPT in reducing decision uncertainty and women's attitude to choice of birthing positions. The objectives of the DCS were: (1) to evaluate the psychometric properties of a DCS that elicits women's uncertainty in making a health-related decision – in this case, the choice from eight birthing positions; (2) to identify factors contributing to the uncertainty; and (3) to elicit women's perceptions of the efficacy of their decision-making in relation to choice of birthing position.

No significant differences were found in the way that women made a decision on birth position with regard to ease of making their choice. However, women in the control group were significantly more unsure ($P<0.05$) about what to do following the decision, compared with women in the experimental group. This suggests that women in the experimental group were more certain about how to make their choices known to the midwives caring for them in labour. This became evident when women in the experimental group identified that they were significantly clearer that the choice they had made was the best choice for them ($P<0.05$).

The concept of choice introduces a degree of uncertainty, for unless women are given the information they need to make a choice, uncertainty in the decision process is inevitable. This was clear from the findings for the control and experimental groups. The experimental group was given a focused course of information on the pros and cons of each of the eight positions on offer. They were also informed about the evidence for and against the use of each position, advised on how to go about making their choices known to the midwives, and tips on how to adopt upright positions in labour and how to practise using each position at home in preparation for labour. The intensive 75-minute session was intended to familiarise and empower women to make a decision to deliver in the upright position if they so wished. It is clear from the findings that women in the experimental group were indeed empowered to be explicit about their choices, and were more certain about the choices they had made, compared with the control group.

Significantly more women in the control group than the experimental group (P<0.025) indicated that they felt the need for more information. This demonstrates that the intensive, focused session had significantly influenced women's cognitive thought in terms of the degree of knowledge they possessed.

Information represents power (Weaver, 1998). Knowledge is a powerful resource, and equipping women with sufficient knowledge empowers them to exercise that knowledge. When women are in labour, they are at their most vulnerable. Women who possess sufficient knowledge to be confident about what they want would, in turn, have control over their childbirth. In this sense, the findings show that choice and control are synonymous.

The findings show that significantly more women in the experimental group than the control group (P<0.01) disagreed that the last trimester of their pregnancy was too soon for them to make a decision on birth positions. This suggests that women who were empowered with the knowledge of birth positions were more decisive.

Both groups of women were pleased to have the opportunity to make a decision on their choice of position before they went into labour. However, significantly more women in the experimental group agreed or strongly agreed with being given the opportunity to make the decision (109 experimental *vs* 81 controls; P<0.025). This highlights again the importance of choice and the emphasis that women place on being given an option to choose their delivery position before going into labour.

This issue can sometimes be underestimated by midwives. In a study of midwife and client relationships, Stapleton (1997) found that ambivalence and negative attitudes of health professionals can affect women's ability to even consider their options. If midwives have a negative or ambivalent attitude towards discussing options and choice with the women in their care, they would be less inclined to discuss the benefits of the upright birthing position. This point was also demonstrated in this study, which found that midwives who were not in favour of using the upright position were less likely to discuss the benefits of its use (see Chapter 9). Stapleton (1997) points out that making options available to the women requires a conscious and deliberate act on the part of the midwife to encourage participation and impart a sense of personal authority towards the women in her care. Failure to do so would inevitably discourage participation and reduce the woman's sense of personal autonomy, thereby disempowering her.

The importance of giving women focused knowledge was further highlighted by the finding that significantly more women in the control group than the experimental group were uncertain about the benefits of using the upright position (P<0.001). Not surprisingly, significantly more women in the same group were unclear about their choice of birth position (P<0.05). In addition, women from both groups wished to be reminded about using upright birthing positions during labour, thus emphasising to midwives the importance of reinforcing the use of upright birthing positions during labour.

Midwives often assume that women will change their minds about their pre-labour decision when they go into labour. However, this study has shown that significantly more women in the experimental group agreed or strongly agreed that they would stick with their decision when they were in labour (P<0.005), implying that they were unlikely to change their minds. This demonstrates the powerful influence of focused information on women's ability to make a firm decision.

Further support for the value of informed choice is provided by the finding that significantly more women in the experimental group than the control group identified that they had made an informed choice regarding their preferences for birth positions (P<0.005).

Value of focused information on decision-making

Significantly more women in the experimental group felt that the decision they made regarding choice of birthing position was the best decision possible for them (P<0.01). This highlights the value of focused information in increasing certainty in decision-making.

Focused information also had a positive effect on women's decision-making in relation to other issues, such as choice of pain relief. For example, significantly more women (P<0.005) in the experimental group felt that they would stick with their choice of pain relief compared with women in the control group, who were less certain about their decision. This finding is surprising, given that women from the control group received more information about choice of pain relief than women in the experimental group.

Following delivery, women were asked to complete a post-delivery questionnaire. No significant differences were found in the birth delivery outcome: 61% of women in the control group and 60% in the experimental group had a normal delivery. Further analysis showed the true rate to be 67% and 64% respectively, as more women from the experimental group underwent caesarean section, although the differences were not significant.

More women from the experimental group identified the value of the educational session in helping them to focus on their choice of position during the second stage of labour, although the difference between the groups was not significant. The findings revealed that, in most cases (42% of the control group, 44% of the experimental group), midwives made the final decision on the choice of birth position. This suggests that women were disempowered during the second stage of labour. It demonstrates that midwives are in a position of power when they are caring for women, and can reduce a woman's level of control by not bowing to her choice, leaving her feeling 'dispossessed' by the knowledge and control she thought she had.

In addition, not all women who were certain about the choices they made through the possession of knowledge would necessarily have their choice met by the midwives. This was shown by the finding that less than half the women (44%) from the experimental group and just over a third (34%) from the control group actually delivered in their pre-determined position of choice. It may be that some women need reassurance and permission from the midwives, despite being given focused information on birthing positions. Walters and Kirkham (1997) pointed out that 'the feedback of information to mothers was in the control of professionals'.

These findings reinforce the view that midwives have the power to control the labour process, and can easily deprive, disempower and disregard women by not relinquishing control to them. Indeed, the extent to which women are given control over their decision-making can often be controlled by midwives, for they can select the choices available to the women in their care (Mander, 1993) and the information they give the women. This issue is particularly worrying, as the findings show that most women (77%) agreed strongly or very strongly that they would like to be reminded about the benefits of upright positions when they go into labour. Moreover, significantly more women (P<0.005) in the experimental group were also certain that they would stick to their decision on their choice of birth position, yet a third of the women were not able to collaborate with their midwife on their decision.

The findings do not support the hypothesis that women who receive focused information on using the upright position would proceed to use it for delivery; however, the ease of decision-making and negotiation between the women and the midwives was more apparent in the group that received focused information (experimental group). The finding that significantly more women in the experimental group were able to use the upright position in the first stage of labour (P<0.025) supports the hypothesis that focused information is of value in helping women with their decision-making during this stage of labour. Focused information was also found to be significantly more effective than general information in helping women collaborate more easily with the midwife during labour (P<0.001). However, more than a third (37%) of the women were not able to collaborate with their midwife on their decision about the choice of position during delivery.

Midwives' role and power – who makes the decisions in labour?

Results showed that midwives controlled the birth process during the second stage of labour. This was reinforced by the finding that most midwives used directive pushing (56% control group *vs* 42% experimental group), which meant that they controlled how and when women should push, compared with indirect pushing (18% control group *vs* 25% experimental group), where women had full control over the pushing and pushed only when the urge or desire to push was apparent. Yet numerous studies have shown that the directive method of pushing is ill advised, as it lengthens the second stage of labour (Caldeyro-Barcia, 1979a, 1979b) and reduces blood flow to the uterus and lower limbs (Bassell et al, 1980). Studies have also identified an increase in the incidence of fetal heart rate abnormality (Knauth and Haloburdo, 1986), delay in the progress of labour and increased incidence of instrumental delivery with directive pushing (McQueen and Mylrea, 1977; Maresh et al, 1983). Moreover, Thomson (1993) found a negative correlation between length of the second stage and venous cord blood pH at delivery in the directed pushing group, compared with the spontaneous or indirect pushing group, in whom there was no negative correlation.

The findings suggest that midwives in the current study were not putting theory into practice in relation to the evidence from these studies. This may reflect the fact that most of the midwives were not up to date with current knowledge, as suggested by the finding that the majority of the midwives only read one professional journal regularly. The findings support the view that current traditional practice in relation to use of the semi-recumbent birthing position, the method of pushing and the way that midwives appear to take control over the childbirth process is in part due to their lack of evidence-based knowledge or their inability to find time to read, and therefore to process and assimilate, the evidence-based information. However, despite evidence that midwives appeared to have more control over the women, the majority of the midwives (75%) stated that they were able to discuss the method of pushing with the mother. This suggests that the women experienced a degree of disempowerment: on the one hand, midwives felt that they discussed decision-making with the women; on the other hand, they took control over decision-making with respect to pushing.

Similarities were found in other areas of decision-making. For example, although the majority of the women collaborated with the midwife during the first stage of labour, a quarter of the women did not have the opportunity to discuss the choice of delivery position with the midwife, again reflecting the shift in power between the mother and the midwife; it may be that the women themselves could not control the situation. Green et al (1990a) proposed that a woman's desire for control was often different in emergency and non-emergency situations, thereby rationalising why women appeared more in control during the first stage of labour, which may be seen as a non-emergency situation, and less in control during the second stage, which may appear to them to be an emergency situation requiring the midwife's expertise. They were therefore more willing to relinquish control by that stage. This is supported by the finding in the current trial that most women were satisfied with their choice of delivery position even though they did not end up using their position of choice.

There appeared to be an association between midwife's preference for a particular birthing position and the actual position adopted by the women at delivery. Of the top four birthing positions used by the women (recumbent, semi-recumbent, left lateral and kneeling), the semi-recumbent, left lateral and kneeling positions were identified by the midwives as their highest preference. The evidence suggests that midwives were more likely to deliver in a position that reflected their own preference than one that reflected the woman's preference. It was found that midwives played a significant role in women's choice of birthing positions and that, irrespective of how much collaboration, cooperation or discussion took place, midwives' preference for birthing positions appeared to supersede women's own preference during the second stage of labour.

In addition, comments from mothers revealed that some women had difficulty in collaborating with their midwife, for example:

> '...due to being strapped to the monitor for the last hour of the 1st stage.'

> 'I couldn't be in the position I wanted, which was the standing position. and this was very frustrating...'

Collaborative decision-making

The importance of collaborative decision-making should not be underestimated. Few midwives would argue against the need to collaborate with the women in their care in every aspect of care delivery. In the current trial, women in the experimental group found it easier to collaborate with the midwives, compared with women in the control group. This may be due to the increased empowerment afforded the women by the focused educational session; increased empowerment was less apparent in the control group.

Effective collaboration requires a dynamic, flexible and non-hierarchical approach to care, and the effort of more than one person to accomplish a mutually determined goal (Bailes and Jackson, 2000). It is therefore not only a necessary process but also one that requires a certain amount of skill and acknowledgement from the midwife, because it involves relinquishing control and transferring power to the women. The term 'collaboration' conjures up an image of sharing; within midwifery practice it involves the sharing of information, knowledge, and power. However, effective collaboration is only accomplished through good communicative practices, mutual trust, respect and interdependence (Bailes and Jackson, 2000); it is a process of give and take in the context of a changing balance of power (Ivey et al, 1988; Stichler, 1995; Keleher, 1998; Stapleton, 1998). It is important that the balance of power tips in favour of the women in the context of labour, when women are at their most vulnerable.

The findings suggest that, for some women, collaborative decision-making existed only during the early stages of labour, and that midwives took control of the decision-making process during the second stage of labour. In a sense, the collaborative decision effort became a 'controlled decision effort' when midwives were controlling the labour process. For collaboration to succeed, not only must all those involved in the decision-making process be willing to acknowledge their limitations, differences, strengths and weaknesses and have their own sense of autonomy (Bailes and Jackson, 2000), but there must also be a heightened sense of mutual cooperation, active participation and engaging communication between the midwife and the women. Positive collaboration can only benefit women in labour, even though the collaborative process may not result in women achieving their ultimate choice of position. This was evident in the women who identified that they were able to collaborate with the midwife even though they did not end up with their initial choice of birth position. It would appear that just being given the opportunity to collaborate with the midwife was sufficient for some women; for others, factors such as being looked after by a caring midwife or one willing to cooperate with the women also influenced their preferences. This was evident in the reasons provided by the women for not giving birth in their preferred position, such as:

> *'I collaborated with the midwife but did not end up with my initial choice because I was just too tired.'*

> *'The midwife was very cooperative, even though I did not end up using the kneeling position...but I managed to discuss it with her.'*

> *'The labour was too quick to maintain the position of my choice, but I managed to point out my preference to the midwife, whom I am sure would have gone along with my decision if I insisted.'*

These comments suggest that the women gained a sense of satisfaction and mutual worth with the midwife during the collaborative process. Such a sense of caring for one another was also identified by Stapleton (1998) in a study on the collaborative benefits of team-building, and by Ivey et al (1988), who highlighted the effectiveness of collaborative decision-making between physicians and nurses in healthcare settings. Keleher (1998) found that when practitioners devote time, energy and attention to the collaborative process, the participants develop a sense of caring for one another, and the collaborative relationship is increased. Indeed, this is a form of 'confidence-building', which can only enhance the relationship between midwives and the women in their care.

In contrast, failure to communicate, and non-meaningful interactions such as ignoring and not listening to one another, are barriers to collaborative practice (McLain, 1988). Such behaviour may also occur between midwives and women when collaborative decision-making is poor. Examples include selective listening, midwives failing to reinforce information, or lack of collaboration, as evident in the following comments from mothers:

> 'The first midwife I had did not make me feel very comfortable and did not discuss the various options.'

> 'My midwife did not discuss birth positions with me; I had to ask ... in the end she did not really listen...'

> 'Decisions and options need to be made and considered before labour, as time is needed to communicate with the midwife the options, and the midwife needs to respect individual wishes.'

> 'It was nice to discuss with the midwife, but when they change shifts it seemed that they hadn't communicated, for example, husband cutting the cord, position preferences etc.'

Other barriers to effective collaborative decision-making include educational differences, gender issues, hierarchical relationships, social class and economics (Sheer, 1996). Issues generated by the women in the trial also highlighted differences in the philosophy of choice. What midwives wanted for women was not the same as what women thought they needed for themselves, as evident from the following comments:

> 'I wanted to use the upright position, but the midwife said that I couldn't but gave no reasons.'

> 'One midwife allowed me to adopt any position and used the Sonicaid; another said that I had to be monitored and I ended up on the bed.'

> 'I was in early labour and I wanted my husband to be with me...but once I was transferred down to the wards ... my husband was sent home without any discussion with me.'

It is worthy of note that, although most women collaborated with their midwife and did not achieve their desired choice of birthing position, 68% were nevertheless satisfied with their decision on birth positions. This is because, for some women, as long as they were able to adopt an upright position, it did not matter that their particular choice was not met. However, it is important to remember that some women from the experimental group and the control group were not able to collaborate with their midwife on their choice of position at delivery, and this had an effect on their overall satisfaction. The benefits of collaborative decision-making have been demonstrated in this trial, and in numerous other studies (Ivey et al, 1988; Rothman, 1991; Izzo, 1994; Keleher, 1998; Stapleton, 1998; Goer, 1999; Lavender et al, 1999; Bailes and Jackson, 2000). It is a pertinent issue that midwives need to address. Perhaps the question here is not whether collaborative decision-making took place, but what followed from the collaborative effort. In other words, it is not so much the quantity of the collaboration but the quality of the collaborative effort that is at stake.

The importance of being fully informed about any decision that is to be made while in labour was highlighted by most of the women in the study. The findings concur with other studies showing that labouring women desire as much information as possible (Garcia, 1982; Ley, 1982; Niven, 1992; Coppen, 1994; Quine and Rutter, 1996; O'Cathain et al, 2002; Wood, 2003). In a classic observation study that looked at information giving and communication by midwives in a group of 113 women, Kirkham (1989) found that information was what they wanted most from midwives.

Women's comments at the end of the postnatal questionnaire highlighted three themes. The first was the value of an educational session on women's decision-making, which in turn empowered them to collaborate with midwives on their choice of birthing position. Examples of these comments are:

> *'I found seeing you in labour very helpful as I was able to be more assertive with the midwife.'*

> *'Your advice on using the birth ball was very good for the length of labour and I was able to try all the positions recommended.'*

In contrast, the second theme identified the difficulties that some women experienced in making a decision during labour. Examples include: difficulty due to the pain experienced in labour; technological barriers, such as monitoring; insertion of infusions; and, more worryingly, breakdown in communication between the women and the midwife.

The third theme was concerned with the impact of the unpredictability of labour on decision-making. For example, some women had a quick labour and found it impossible to make any decision during labour. Another felt that there was a need to go with the flow of labour, and the unpredictability of labour made decision-making difficult. These comments suggest that, although most women found the focused information invaluable, other factors, such as the need to be monitored and barriers to communication, affected their decision-making process. In addition, the unpredictability of labour also had an impact on their ability to make any decision during labour.

Conclusion

Overall, therefore, the findings highlight the effectiveness of providing focused information on birthing positions to women. Effectiveness in terms of women's increased knowledge of birthing positions, certainty about their choice of birthing position and their ability to collaborate and communicate with the midwife was significantly more apparent in the experimental group than the control group. However, the findings also showed that the midwife controlled the decision-making process during the second stage of labour and that women were not able to focus on their choice of birthing position during the second stage of labour. However, this was not the case during the first stage of labour.

The findings can be interpreted in two ways. First, it could be argued that midwives felt that they needed to take over decision-making during the second stage because the women were unable to focus on their choice of birthing position. Second, and paradoxically, it could be that women were unable to focus on their choice of birthing position because midwives were not reinforcing or empowering them with their choice of position.

Finally, the findings highlight the importance of focused information to collaborative decision-making between the woman and the midwife during labour. In this study, although focused information did not influence the rate of normal delivery, it did have a significant effect in the first stage of labour as significantly more women in the experimental group adopted upright birthing positions. The findings therefore do support the hypothesis that focused information is effective in increasing knowledge levels, in reducing decisional conflict and enhancing decision certainty with respect to women's choice of birthing position, and in promoting collaborative decision-making during labour, particularly the first stage.

Contribution to the body of knowledge

The research discussed in this book has contributed to the body of knowledge and added to the evidence base for midwifery care, by addressing women's views of the childbirth process in relation to birthing positions.

The primary study was a randomised controlled trial (RCT). This was an original attempt to investigate women's preferences regarding birthing positions by introducing an intervention (focused information) to assist women in the decision-making process. The importance of informed choice, the process of decision-making, and women's preferences for different birthing positions were highlighted. The RCT is considered the 'gold standard' of research, and this RCT is the first to evaluate the effectiveness of focused information on women's decision-making regarding birthing positions. Double-blinding of the trial meant that it provides the most reliable evidence about the relative effectiveness of 'focused education' on the decision-making process between the participants (women) and the care-providers (midwives).

The results of the study support the hypothesis that focused information is effective in increasing level of knowledge and reducing decisional conflict, highlighting the importance of providing informed choice to women. The findings concur with the views of the *Changing Childbirth* Report (Department of Health, 1993), the *National Service Framework for Children, Young People and Maternity Services* (Department of Health, 2004, 2005) and the World Health Organization (1996), which recommended that women should be informed of all available choices in childbirth. It also supports the view that focused information will ease the decision process for women and empower them with the confidence to collaborate with the midwife on their decision to use the upright position in labour.

Encouraging women to deliver in the upright position through the use of focused information supports the findings of the systematic reviews of Coppen (2002) and Gupta and Nikodem (2000a) that upright positions during labour and delivery are more beneficial to women than recumbent positions. It also identifies with Hanson's (1998) and Walsh's (1998, 1999) studies, which demonstrated the value of increasing midwives' knowledge of birthing positions in promoting the use of upright positions in labour. Perhaps improving communication channels between midwives and women and the need to change practice attitudes are the real issues, and the key to successfully motivating midwives to change the way they practise.

Finally, the findings of this study could have many implications for the future of midwifery practice. For example, the results suggest that cost-effectiveness could be improved by replacing the general parent education session by a more focused education session. Another innovation could be the setting up of 'midwifery consultation' sessions in the antenatal period to meet the individual needs of mothers who are uncertain about the choices available to them. These sessions could be extended to include other issues in pregnancy and childbirth, such as place of birth, induction of labour, the controversial use of continuous fetal monitoring and pain relief in labour. This could be achieved by the use of ADAPT, a decision-making instrument that is easily modified to suit different decision needs, which midwives can be taught to apply in practice.

Such innovative practice could become particularly important in today's climate of increasing litigation (Dingwall, 1993; Dimond, 1997, 2001) and pressure to conform with government initiatives, as the sessions would be based on the use of current best available evidence to help women to make better decisions. This could, in turn, encourage midwives to read more peer-reviewed research-based journals and keep pace with evidence-based research in midwifery practice. In addition, it may lead to midwives encouraging women to deliver in upright positions, thereby increasing the use of upright positions in labour, and the transfer of theoretical knowledge into evidence-based clinical practice.

Appendixes

APPENDIX 1: The ADAPT decision instrument – developed by Regina Coppen

Please read the whole question before answering.

Do not hesitate to ask me to clarify anything that you do not understand.

Part 1: CHOICE OF BIRTH POSITIONS

1. Following the seminar, please rate how much you know about the different birthing positions for delivery:

```
0 ----------------- 3 ----------------- 5 ----------------- 8 ----------------- 10
nothing        a little        some            a lot        almost
                            knowledge                    everything
```

2. Please give a rating against **all** the 8 possible delivery positions listed below by scoring any number from 0–100% in each of the boxes. This will help me to compare how much you like one preference over another. For example, if you like the kneeling position most, as your first choice you should give this the highest scoring percentage. The position you would not wish to use at all should be rated as 0% and those you like the least would have the lowest scores.

Key guidelines to each percentage:

0–19%	Very weak preference
20–39%	Weak preference
40–59%	No preference for any position (neutral)
60–79%	Strong preference
80–100%	Very strong preference

Preference is defined as your liking, predisposition or partiality towards the use of this particular delivery position

Recumbent (flat in bed)	⬚	Squatting	⬚
Semi-recumbent (sitting up with pillows or a wedge 45° or less)	⬚	Semi-squatting (Supported squat)	⬚
Left lateral	⬚	Standing	⬚
All-fours (hands and knees)	⬚	Kneeling	⬚

3. For your highest scoring preference, can you give reasons why this is your most preferred position? (Tick any which apply)

Tried it at previous birth, and I like it	⬚
Appears the most comfortable	⬚
Influenced by the research studies during the seminar session	⬚
Appears the most natural position	⬚
I am more in control	⬚
None of the above	⬚

▼

Any other reason (please specify) ....

APPENDIX 1 (cont'd): The ADAPT decision instrument developed by Regina Coppen

4. For your highest scoring preference, please identify how important it is for you to be able to use this position for delivery:

Very important
Important
Not so important
Not important at all

5. For the position that you scored the least, please give reasons why this is your least preferred position (tick any which apply):

Tried it at previous birth, and dislike it
Appears the least comfortable
Influenced by the research studies during
   the seminar session
Appears the least natural position
I am less in control
None of the above

▼

Any other reason (please specify) ....

PART 2 CHOICE OF PAIN RELIEF

1. Following the seminar, please rate how much you know about pain relief in labour:

0 ------------------ 3 ------------------ 5 ----------------- 8 ------------------ 10
  nothing   a little   some knowledge   a lot   almost everything

2. Please rate your choice of pain relief on a scale of 1–10 by marking against the line which is most appropriate for you:

1. Relaxation techniques   1 -------------------------- 5 -------------------------- 10
                                 least   can't decide   definite choice

2. Water-bath   1 -------------------------- 5 -------------------------- 10
                                 least   can't decide   definite choice

3. TENS   1 -------------------------- 5 -------------------------- 10
                                 least   can't decide   definite choice

4. Entonox   1 -------------------------- 5 -------------------------- 10
                                 least   can't decide   definite choice

5. Pethidine   1 -------------------------- 5 -------------------------- 10
                               least   can't decide   definite choice

6. Epidural   1 -------------------------- 5 -------------------------- 10
                               least   can't decide   definite choice

Please check this questionnaire again to ensure you have not left any questions out.

Name: .... Expected date of delivery: ....

Thank you for completing this questionnaire and for your active participation in this study. Best wishes for the rest of your pregnancy, birth and post-delivery care.

APPENDIX 2: Pre-intervention questionnaire for mothers

CODE NO: [ ]

Section 1: General Information about You and Your Pregnancy

Please tick your answers in the box

NAME: ....

1. Is this your [First] [Second] [Third or more] baby?

2. How old will you be when your baby is due?

18 or less	[ ]
19–25	[ ]
26–35	[ ]
36–40	[ ]
41 or above	[ ]

3. To ensure that we meet the needs of all ethnic groups, we should like to ask you how you think of yourself:

White		[ ]
Black	– African	[ ]
	– Caribbean	
Asian	– Indian	[ ]
	– Pakistani	
	– Bangladeshi	
	– Chinese	[ ]
	– Vietnamese	
	Other (please specify)	

Any other (please specify) ....

4. Please identify your highest educational attainment:

Up to Year 10/11	[ ]
GCSE	
GCE O Level	
A Level	
Diploma	
Degree/Masters	
PhD	

Any other (please specify) ....

Section 2: Your Views on Different Positions in Labour

1. Have you read or heard about the different types of positions that you can try to deliver your baby?

Yes [ ]   No [ ] ➡ go to Question 3

2. If you answer Yes to Question 1, please specify where you have heard about this information (tick any which apply)

APPENDIX 2 (cont'd): Pre-intervention questionnaire for mothers

Parent education classes ☐
NCT classes ☐
Midwife-antenatal check-up ☐
Books or magazines ☐
Media ☐

3. On a scale of 0–10, please rate how much you know about the different positions you can choose to deliver your baby?

0 ----------------- 3 ------------------ 5 ----------------- 8 ----------------- 10
nothing   a little   some   a lot   everything
                            knowledge

4. Have you thought about a particular position to deliver your baby at this stage of your pregnancy?

Yes ☐   No ☐ → Go to Question 5

5. Can you specify which position you would like to deliver your baby?
   (Tick no more than 3 only)

   (1) Recumbent (flat in bed on your back)

   (2) Semi-recumbent (sitting up with pillows or wedge on the bed at 30° or less)

   (3) Left lateral (lying on your side)   (4) Standing

   (5) Squatting   (6) Semi-squatting (between squatting and standing with hands on thighs or suspended with support

   (7) All-fours (hands and knees)   (8) Kneeling

6. Do you have any position you would definitely NOT wish to adopt for delivery? (Tick any which apply)

   YES ☐ **(please specify the number from the list above)** ....

   or NO ☐

Section 3: Your Views on Choice of Pain Relief in Labour

1. How many different choices of pain relief have you heard about in this pregnancy? (Tick any which apply)

   Psychoprophylaxis (relaxation techniques) ☐

   Transcutaneous electrical nerve stimulation (TENS) ☐

   Pethidine ☐

   Entonox ('gas and air') ☐

   Epidural ☐

APPENDIX 2 (cont'd): Pre-intervention questionnaire for mothers

2. On a scale of 0–10, please rate how much you know about pain relief in labour:

0 ------------------ 3 ------------------ 5 ------------------ 8 ------------------ 10
nothing   a little   some   a lot   everything
knowledge

3. Have you thought about a pain relief you would like to try when you are in labour?

Yes ☐ ➡ Please specify from the above list ....

No ☐

Can't decide ☐

Section 4: This Section is about Labour Support

1. Have you thought about having someone to support you in labour?   **Yes / No / Not sure**

2. If you answered Yes, please specify from the list below:

Husband/Partner ☐

A relative ☐

A friend ☐

3. With reference to the choice of position and pain relief, would you like the midwife to make the decision for you in labour? **Please tick your responses.**

Options	Definitely Yes	Yes, only if I can't decide	Definitely No	Not sure
Pain relief				
Position in labour				

I would appreciate it very much if you can give me your response to my invitation as soon as possible. Please tick the relevant box below:

Yes, I would like to attend the seminar: ☐

Please contact me on .... during the day / evening (please specify)

No, I can't attend the seminar, but will be happy to complete any questionnaire for this study ☐

No, I do not wish to participate because: ....

It will help to know why you do not wish to participate for research purposes.

Thank you for completing the questionnaire. Kindly post it in the stamped addressed envelope provided.

APPENDIX 3: The Decisional Conflict scale

Decisional Conflict Scale

Now, thinking about the choices you have just made, please look at the following comments some people make when deciding about choices in labour.

Please show how strongly you agree or disagree with these comments by CIRCLING THE NUMBER from 1 (strongly agree) to 5 (strongly disagree) that best shows how you feel about the decision you have just made on pain relief and birthing positions:

	Strongly agree	Agree	Neither agree nor disagree	Disagree	Strongly disagree
Decision uncertainty					
The decision on **birth position** is hard for me to make	1	2	3	4	5
I'm unsure what to do in this decision	1	2	3	4	5
It's clear what choice is best for me	1	2	3	4	5
The decision on **pain relief** is hard for me to make	1	2	3	4	5
I'm sure what to do in this decision	1	2	3	4	5
It's clear what choice is best for me	1	2	3	4	5
Factors contributing to uncertainty					
I'm aware of the choices I have on different positions in labour	1	2	3	4	5
I feel I know the benefits of upright positions for delivery	1	2	3	4	5
I need more information and advice about the choices on birth positions	1	2	3	4	5
I need more information and advice about the choices on pain relief	1	2	3	4	5
It would help me to be reminded about the benefits of upright positions when I am in labour	1	2	3	4	5
I know how important the benefits are to me in this decision	1	2	3	4	5
It's hard to decide if the benefits of upright positions are more important to me than the conventional mode of delivery	1	2	3	4	5
I feel pressure from others in making this decision	1	2	3	4	5

Please turn over the page:

APPENDIX 3 (cont'd): The Decisional Conflict scale

	Strongly agree	Agree	Neither agree nor disagree	Disagree	Strongly disagree
I have the right amount of support from others in making this decision	1	2	3	4	5
I feel it is too soon for me to make a decision on choice of **birth positions**	1	2	3	4	5
I am pleased to be given the choice to make this decision before I go into labour	1	2	3	4	5
I feel it is too soon for me to make a decision on choice of **pain relief**	1	2	3	4	5
I am pleased to be given the choice to make this decision before I go into labour	1	2	3	4	5

Perceived effective decision-making with reference to BIRTH POSITIONS

I feel I have made an informed choice	1	2	3	4	5
My decision shows what is most important	1	2	3	4	5
I expect to stick with my decision	1	2	3	4	5
The decision I made was the best decision possible for me personally	1	2	3	4	5
I am satisfied that my decision was consistent with my personal values	1	2	3	4	5
I am satisfied that this was my decision to make	1	2	3	4	5
I am satisfied with my decision	1	2	3	4	5

Perceived effective decision-making with reference to PAIN RELIEF

I feel I have made an informed choice	1	2	3	4	5
My decision shows what is most important	1	2	3	4	5
I expect to stick with my decision	1	2	3	4	5
I am satisfied that my decision was consistent with my personal values	1	2	3	4	5
I am satisfied that this was my decision to make	1	2	3	4	5
I am satisfied with my decision	1	2	3	4	5

Thank you for completing the questionnaire.

Adapted from O'Connor A (1995) Validation of a decisional conflict scale. *Medical Decision Making* 15(1): 25-29; Homes-Rovner M, Kroll J, et al (1996) Patient satisfaction with health care decisions. *Medical Decision Making* 16(1): 58-64

APPENDIX 4: Post-delivery questionnaire for mothers

POST-DELIVERY QUESTIONNAIRE FOR MOTHERS

Name ....

CONGRATULATIONS ON THE BIRTH OF YOUR BABY!

Thank you for agreeing to complete this form

1. Did you have a normal delivery? Yes/No ➤ If No, please specify ....

Please note: Please complete this form to the end as far as possible whether you had a normal delivery or not as it is still relevant to the study. Thank you

2. What delivery position did you have your baby? Please tick one only

Lying flat on the bed	Sitting up on the bed	Lying on my side (lateral)
Standing	Squatting	Semi-squatting
Hands & knees (on all-fours)	Kneeling	

In this section, please mark X against the percentage closest to your answer or tick as appropriate

3. Did you have any preference for a particular birth position during the course of labour?
   Yes / No ➤ If no, skip question 4 and go straight to question 5 onwards

4. Did you deliver in the position of your choice? Yes / No ➤ If No, can you think of reasons?

   ....

5. With reference to the session you attended, did it help you to make a decision to use upright positions during the first stage of labour? (First stage is defined from the start of regular contractions to when you are ready to push baby out)

   0% ---------------------- 25% ---------------------- 50% ------------------------- 75% -------------------- 100%
   unhelpful   helped a little   moderately helpful   helped alot   very helpful

6. With reference to the session you attended, did it help you to make a decision to focus on your choice to use upright position for the actual delivery of the baby?

   0% ---------------------- 25% ---------------------- 50% ------------------------- 75% -------------------- 100%
   unhelpful   helped a little   moderately helpful   helped alot   very helpful

7. Were you able to collaborate your decision about which position to use for delivery with the midwife who looked after you in labour? Yes / No ➤ If No, please go to question 7 (1.3)

   Yes 1.1: I was able to use my pre-determined position of choice
        1.2: Midwife and I collaborated but I did not end up with my choice of position

   Please describe how this final position was decided? ....

APPENDIX 4 (cont'd): Post-delivery questionnaire for mothers

QUESTION 7 (1.3) or No, I was not able to collaborate my decision about which position to use for delivery with the midwife who looked after me in labour:

If No, please give reasons:
Because (circle any of the reasons that apply):

1.3   I have not made any decision about a delivery position
1.4:   There was no opportunity with the midwife
1.5:   My labour was too quick
1.6:   I did not think about my choice of position at the time
1.7:   I was happy for my midwife to decide
1.8:   I was unsure which position to use, so my midwife made the decision anyway
1.9:   My midwife/doctor (delete as appropriate) made the decision for me to deliver on the bed
2.0:   I made the decision to deliver on the bed
2.1:   I had epidural analgesia by choice
2.2:   I was advised to have epidural
2.3:   I was monitored continuously and had to lie on the bed
2.4:   I changed my mind about my birth position from the original decision
2.5:   Other reasons – please specify: ....

8. Would you have liked to be given more time to make your decision about which position to use for delivery while in labour?

Yes, definitely   Yes, possibly   No, not really   Don't know

9. Did the educational session help you to collaborate with your midwife more easily?

Yes, definitely   Yes, possibly   No, not really   Don't know

10. Thinking back on your birth experience, how satisfied were you with the decision that was made on your birth position? (Please mark an X on a scale of 0–100%)

0% -------------------- 25% ------------------ 50% -------------------- 75% ----------------------- 100%
very dissatisfied   dissatisfied   satisfied   mostly satisfied   very satisfied

11. Thinking back on the particular session you attended, would you find such educational sessions useful in helping you to make informed decisions about other issues in pregnancy or labour?

Yes, definitely   Yes, possibly   No, not really   Don't know

12. How important is it to you to be fully informed about any decisions that is to be made while in labour?

Very important   Important   Quite important   Not important at all

13. Would you like to add any further comments here about decision-making in labour?

THANK YOU VERY MUCH FOR TAKING TIME TO COMPLETE THIS QUESTIONNAIRE Kindly post it in the SAE provided

---

APPENDIX 5: Questionnaire to establish midwives' views on birthing positions

RESEARCH ON DELIVERY POSITION: QUESTIONNAIRE FOR MIDWIVES

Please be assured that confidentiality will be maintained at all times. Your name will not be identified and it is only used for the purpose of the research analysis.
Please enter your name or password. If you prefer to use a password, please remember to use the same password when completing the post-delivery sheet each time.

Name or Password: ....

1) Do you work mainly in the Delivery suite / Community / Postnatal / Antenatal?

2) How long have you been allocated to this area? (Please tick)

Less than 3 months		1–2 years	
4–6 months		3–5 years	
7–12 months		5 years or more	

3) Length of experience as a practising midwife:

1–2 years		5–7 years		>10 years	
2–4 years		8–10 years			

4) Have you ever attended any educational session on delivery positions ?

Yes (please state approximately how long ago)   ....

No [ ]   Can't remember [ ]

5) PLEASE READ THIS QUESTION CAREFULLY:

Please rate your personal preference for each **delivery** position by scoring 0–100% against the degree of preference for each position **you would use**. For example, your least preferred position would have the lowest score and the position you prefer most would be given the highest score.

Preference is defined as your liking, predisposition or partiality towards the use of this particular position as a midwife.

Recumbent (flat in bed) [ ]	Squatting [ ]
Semi-recumbent (lying 30° or less) [ ]	Semi-squatting [ ] (between squatting and standing, both hands on thighs or suspended with support)
Lateral [ ]	Standing [ ]
Lithotomy [ ]	Kneeling [ ]
All-fours (hands and knees) [ ]	Other (specify) ....

APPENDIX 5 (cont'd): Questionnaire to establish midwives' views on birthing positions

6) For your highest scoring preference, how often would you use this position for delivery?
   Tick one box only:

   All of the time ☐   Most of the time ☐

   Some of the time ☐   None of the time ☐

7) Can you give reasons why this is your most preferred position?

   ....

   ....

8) For the position that you scored the least, please give reasons why this is your least preferred position?

   ....

   ....

9) If the women you are caring for wish to deliver in a position you are **not experienced** with, would you do it anyway?

   Yes, definitely ☐

   Yes, but only with the help of an experienced midwife ☐

   No ☐

   Comment, if any:

   ....

10) If the women you are caring for wish to deliver in a position you are **experienced** with, but **do not feel comfortable** with, would you do it anyway?

    Yes, definitely ☐   No, but may give into pressure from the women ☐

    Yes, possibly ☐   No, but may give into peer pressure ☐

    Definitely not, regardless of women's wishes ☐

    Comment, if any:

    ....

11) In your professional opinion, excluding all caesarean, forceps, ventouse, epidural cases, why do most women deliver their baby on the bed in the recumbent or semi-recumbent position?

    ....

12) What professional journals do you read regularly (defined as at least fortnightly)?

    ....

    Thank you for taking the time to complete this form. It is vital to the research and much appreciated
    Please place the sheet in the **'Delivery Position Research Box'** which is kept in the delivery suite, **or if you so wish, post it to: Regina Coppen (address supplied).**

APPENDIX 6: Post-delivery questionnaire for midwives

RESEARCH ON DELIVERY POSITION

POST-DELIVERY QUESTIONNAIRE FOR MIDWIVES TO COMPLETE
Please be assured that confidentiality will be maintained at all times. Your name will not be identified and it is only used for the purpose of research analysis.

Midwife's name ....

Section A: Please complete this sheet at the end of the delivery – Delete appropriate section

Mother's name (very important!) ....

1) **Place of birth:** hospital / home   2) **Baby's date of birth:** ....

3) **Parity:** primipara / multipara

4) **Gestation**: <37 weeks / 37–40 weeks / >40 weeks

5) **Length of labour:** 1st stage .... 2nd stage .... 3rd stage ....

6) **Did the mother adopt different positions in the first stage of labour? Yes / No / Not sure**

   If so, please specify the position/s used: ....

7) What **method of pushing** was used at the second stage? (circle one only)

   (a) Active pushing (directive)   (b) Passive pushing (non-directive)   (c) Both types

8a) Method of delivery (please circle): Normal Yes / No ➤ If No, please go straight to 8b

> **8b)** If Forceps / Ventouse / Caesarean – Please give reasons. Circle any which apply:
>
> Elective / Emergency / Maternal distress / Fetal distress / Delay in 2nd stage /
>
> Other reasons (please specify) ....

Section B (To be completed for normal delivery outcomes only)

1) Where was the mother delivered?   **On the bed / Off the bed**

2) **Specific position used for the actual delivery (please circle one position only):**

   Recumbent (flat in bed)   Semi-recumbent (sitting up with pillows or wedge <45°)

   Lateral   Lithotomy   Squatting   Semi-squatting   Standing

   All-fours (hands and knees)   Kneeling   Any other (please specify) ....

3. Please identify, from the list above, **the different types of positions** that were attempted during the second stage of labour :..

4) **For the delivery position used, please identify who made the final decision:**

   Mother / Midwife / Mother & Midwife / Mother & Partner/ Partner / Obstetrician

5) **Were you able to discuss the choice of delivery position with the mother in labour?**

   Yes / No / Can't remember

6) What **pain relief** was used? ....

7) Total estimated **blood loss** ....

8) **Perineum state** (please circle): Intact/Graze/1st/2nd/3rd degree tear/Episiotomy/Sutured/Not sutured

Thank you very much for taking the time to complete the questionnaire.

APPENDIX 7: Seminar checklist – Experimental group

SEMINAR CHECKLIST – EXPERIMENTAL GROUP

DATE: ....

TIME: ....

ISSUES DISCUSSED	YES	NO	Comments
Welcome – Getting to know each other			
Introduction to the session			
Fears & expectations in pairs/trio			
Group feedback & Coping strategies			
Research evidence: Positions in first stage of labour			
Diagrams of 8 different birthing positions			
Demonstrate with doll and pelvis and action			
Pros and cons of each position			
Early labour tips – at home, support, food & drink			
Pain relief and use of water			
Monitoring in labour			
VIDEO: Delivery in the upright position			
Summary			
Questionnaire to complete			
Handouts: Positions and exercise tips			
Other:			

APPENDIX 8: Seminar checklist – Control group

SEMINAR CHECKLIST – CONTROL GROUP

DATE: ....

TIME: ....

ISSUES DISCUSSED	YES	NO	Comments
Welcome – Getting to know each other			
Introduction to the session			
Fears & expectations in pairs/trio			
Group feedback Coping strategies			
Early labour tips – at home, support, bath			
Use of pain relief			
Pros and cons of pain relief			
Monitoring in labour			
Nutrition and hydration			
Diagram of different positions			
VIDEO: Exercises in pregnancy and Normal delivery			
Summary			
Questionnaire to complete (10 minutes)			
Handouts: Pain relief			
Other:			

Glossary

Anaesthesia: Deadening of sensation.

Anaesthetic: Drug that deadens sensation.

Anterior: Positioned towards the front.

Artificial rupture of the membranes (ARM): Breaking of the bag of waters by the midwife, using a hooked instrument, to speed up or induce labour. This is often carried out in conjunction with an infusion of synthetic oxytocin into the arm to stimulate contractions.

Attrition: A reduction in the number of participants during the course of a study. The withdrawal of more participants from one group than from another can introduce bias and threaten the internal validity of the research.

Bias: Any influence that distorts the results of a research study.

Bivariate analysis: Statistical test in which the summary values from two groups of the same variable, or two variables within a group, are compared.

Blinding: A procedure which ensures that the study participants do not know whether they are in the intervention group or the control group (single blinding); in double blinding, neither the participants nor those caring for them, e.g. doctors, midwives, health carers or researchers, know the allocation.

Breech presentation: The baby who sits bottom down rather than head down in the uterus is said to be in a breech position. Breech births can be quite difficult, and some, though not all, doctors advise delivering breech babies by caesarean section. Often babies sit in the breech position in mid-pregnancy but turn to the head-down position later on.

Caesarean section: Delivery of the fetus through an incision in the uterine wall.

Causal: Relating to a cause; a causal relationship between two variables is one in which changes in the value of one variable cause the other variable to change.

Chi-squared: A statistical test that is calculated as the sum of the squares of observed values minus expected values, divided by the expected values.

Clinical trial: A large-scale experiment designed to test the effectiveness of a clinical treatment or intervention.

Coding: A procedure for transforming raw data into a standardised format for analysis. Coding qualitative data involves identifying recurrent words, concepts or themes.

Cohort: A group of individuals with some characteristics in common.

Confounding factor or variable: A variable, other than the variable(s) under investigation, that is not controlled for and which may distort the results of experimental research.

Content analysis: A procedure for organising narrative, qualitative data into emerging themes and concepts.

Continuous variable: A variable that can take on an infinite range of values along a specific continuum (e.g. weight, height).

Control: Processes employed to hold the conditions under which an investigation is carried out uniform or constant. In a true experimental design, the control group is the group that does not receive the intervention or treatment under investigation. The scores of the dependent variable for the control and the experimental groups are used to evaluate the effect of the independent variable. In other experimental designs, this group may be referred to as the comparison group.

Correlation/correlational: The degree of association between two variables. A tendency for variation in one variable to be linked to variation in a second variable.

Correlation coefficient: A measure of the degree of relationship between two variables. A correlation coefficient lies between +1.0 (indicating a perfect positive relationship), through 0 (indicating no relationship between two variables), to -1.0 (a perfect negative or inverse relationship).

Cronbach's alpha: A statistical test used to assess the reliability of an instrument or tool being tested.

Dependent variable: The outcome measured or the effect in an experimental study. In experimental research, the dependent variable is the variable presumed within the research hypothesis to depend on (be caused by) another variable (the independent variable); it is sometimes referred to as the outcome variable.

Descriptive statistics: Statistical methods used to describe or summarise data collected from a specific sample (e.g. mean, median, mode, range, standard deviation).

Design: The plan of the research, usually in relation to quantitative research.

Dorsal: Pertaining to the back; lying on one's back.

Double-blind trial: A clinical trial in which neither the participants nor the doctors, midwives, health carers or researchers know who is receiving the experimental drug or intervention (experimental group) and who is receiving the placebo or standard comparison treatment (control group). This method is believed to achieve the most accurate, generalisable results because neither the doctors, midwives, health carers or researchers nor the participants can influence the observed results with their psychological biases.

Eclampsia: The convulsive form of pregnancy-induced hypertension; a severe complication of pregnancy.

Efficacy: Strength or potency; effectiveness.

Elective: Non-urgent.

Epidural: An injection of local anaesthetic into the lower back, given for pain relief during labour. This can be topped up via a catheter, which is left in place during labour.

Episiotomy: Incision of the perineum to facilitate delivery and prevent laceration (controversial: studies have shown that it should not to be used routinely to facilitate delivery).

Exclusion criteria: Characteristics that make an individual unsuitable for participation in the research study.

Experimental group: In experimental research, the group of subjects who receive the experimental treatment or intervention under investigation.

Experimental research: A research methodology used to establish cause-and-effect relationships between the independent and dependent variables by manipulation of variables, control and randomisation. A true experiment involves the introduction of a control group (for the purpose of comparison), random allocation of participants to experimental and control groups, and manipulation of the independent variable. Participants are assessed before and after manipulation of the independent variable in order to assess its effect on the dependent variable (the outcome).

Focus group: An interview conducted with a small group of people to explore their ideas on a particular topic.

Forceps delivery: A procedure performed by an obstetrician to expedite delivery when complications arise. An instrument in the shape of a long spoon (forceps) is inserted into the vagina and placed on either side of the baby's head to ease delivery.

Gestation: Pregnancy.

Gravida: A pregnant woman.

Grounded theory: A research approach used to develop conceptual categories/theory about social processes inductively from real-world observations (data) on a selected group of people. The researcher may subsequently make further observations to test the developed categories/theory.

Hawthorne effect: A change that results from the research process and not from the interventions within the research.

Hypothesis: A statement that predicts the relationship between variables (specifically the independent and dependent variables).

Incidence: Number of cases.

Inclusion criteria: The characteristics that determine the suitability of individuals for participation in a study.

Independent variable: The variable (or antecedent) that is assumed to cause or influence the dependent variable(s) or outcome. The independent variable is manipulated in experimental research to observe its effect on the dependent variable(s). It is sometimes referred to as the treatment variable.

Inferential statistics: Statistics designed to allow inference from a sample statistic to a population parameter; commonly used to test hypotheses of similarities and differences in subsets of the sample under study.

Informed consent: Voluntary consent by an individual to participation in a clinical study, based on a full understanding of the possible benefits and risks.

Invasive method: Relating to a medical procedure or intervention by a doctor or health professional, e.g. a nurse.

Labour: The process of expulsion of the fetus from the uterus.

Latent content analysis: A qualitative analysis technique used to classify words in a text into a few categories or themes that are chosen for their theoretical importance. Similar to Content analysis.

Lateral: Towards the side.

Likert scale: A method used to measure attitudes, in which respondents indicate their degree of agreement or disagreement with a series of statements. Scores are summed to give a composite measure of attitudes.

Manipulation: An intervention usually instigated or designed by the researchers, the effects of which are under investigation or study.

Midwife: Meaning 'with woman', pertaining to childbirth; an expert in the field of normal obstetrics/childbirth or midwifery.

Midwifery: The techniques and practice of a midwife, including childbirth assistance, the independent care of essentially normal healthy women and infants before, during and after childbirth, and, in collaboration with medical personnel, the consultation, management and referral of cases in which abnormalities develop.

Method: The tools or technique used to undertake a research study, or all the information needed for other researchers to replicate a study.

Negative correlation: A relationship between two variables where higher values on one variable tend to be associated with lower values on the second variable; sometimes referred to as an inverse relationship.

Nominal level: Lowest level of measurement used when data can be organised into categories that are exclusive and exhaustive but cannot be compared, such as gender, race and marital status.

Non-parametric statistics: Statistical tests that can be used to analyse nominal or ordinal data; they involve less rigorous assumptions than parametric statistics.

Non-significant results/differences: The result of a statistical test which indicates that the outcome of an experimental research study could have occurred through random variation (or chance) at a specified level of significance, rather than as a result of manipulation of the independent variable.

Null hypothesis: A statement that there is no relationship between the independent and dependent variables and that any relationship observed is due to chance or fluctuations in sampling.

Objective: Aim or goal; not influenced by personal feelings or opinions.

Observation: A method of data collection in which data are gathered through visual observations.

Obstetrics: Pertaining to childbirth or midwifery.

Obstetrician: A doctor specialising in the care of women during pregnancy, labour and delivery; expert in the field of abnormal obstetrics/childbirth.

Occipital: The back of the skull.

Occiput: The lower back part of the head.

Ordinal level: Measurement yielding data that can be ranked, but intervals between the ranked data are not necessarily equal, such as levels of coping.

Oxytocin: A hormone secreted by women when they are in labour, which stimulates uterine contractions. When labour is slow, its effect is enhanced by infusion of a synthetic oxytocin (Syntocinon).

P-value: P is the symbol for the probability associated with the outcome of a test of the null hypothesis (i.e. it is the probability that an observed inferential statistic occurred through chance variation). If the P-value is less than or equal to the stated significance level – often set at 5% (P<0.05) or 1% (P<0.01) – the researcher concludes that the results are unlikely to have occurred by chance and are more likely to have occurred because of manipulation of the independent variable; the results are then said to be 'statistically significant'. If the P-value is greater than the significance level, the researcher concludes that the results are likely to have occurred by chance variation, and the results are said to be 'non-significant'.

Parametric statistical analyses: Statistical techniques used when three assumptions are met: (1) sample was drawn from a population for which the variance can be calculated, with normal distribution; (b) level of measurement should be at least interval, with an approximate normal distribution; (3) the data can be treated as random samples.

Parity: The number of pregnancies of a particular woman in which the fetus has reached viability.

Parturition: Giving birth.

Pearson correlation coefficient: A parametric test used to determine relationships among variables. *See* Correlation coefficient

Perineal: Pelvis-related.

Perineum: Area of the body between the anus and the genitals, i.e. between the vagina and the anus in women.

Pilot study: A trial of the research process on a small scale to test the tools and techniques of the study; may also be used to check feasibility, likely recruitment and outcomes.

Placenta: A temporary organ in the womb that allows the fetus to receive nutrients, oxygen and other substances (such as medications) from the mother and to eliminate carbon dioxide and other waste products.

Population: A well-defined group or set that has certain specified properties (e.g. all registered midwives working full-time in Scotland).

Positive correlation: A relationship between two variables where higher values for one variable tend to be associated with higher values for the second variable (e.g. physical activity level and pulse rate).

Posterior: Referring to the back of a structure.

Postpartum: After delivery or childbirth.

Power calculation: The statistical process to calculate the sample size required to achieve statistically significant results in relation to the identified outcome measure of the study.

Primigravida: A woman who is pregnant for the first time.

Prospective study: A study in which data are collected as part of the research process, as opposed to a retrospective study, which uses data already available.

Qualitative data: Information gathered in narrative (non-numeric) form (e.g. the transcript of an unstructured interview).

Quantitative data: Information gathered in numeric form.

Random sampling: A process of selecting a sample whereby each member of the population has an equal chance of being included.

Randomisation: The random assignment of subjects to experimental and control groups (i.e. the allocation to groups is determined by chance).

Randomised controlled trial (RCT): A trial in which participants are randomly assigned to either an intervention group (e.g. focused information, as in this study) or a control group (e.g. general information, as in this study). Both groups are followed up over a specified period of time and the effects of the intervention on specific outcomes (dependent variables) defined at the outset are analysed (e.g. birthing position at delivery).

Range: A measure of variability indicating the difference between the highest and lowest values in a distribution of scores.

Rating scale: Scale that lists an ordered series of categories of a variable and is assumed to be based on an underlying continuum.

Ratio level: A measurement used when the numbers are progressive with identical spacing between each number and there is an absolute zero.

Reliability: The consistency and dependability of a measuring instrument, i.e. an indication of the degree to which it gives the same answers over time, across similar groups and irrespective of who administers it. A reliable measuring instrument will always give the same result on different occasions, assuming that what is being measured has not changed during the intervening period. A number of techniques can be used to ensure the reliability of a standardised measuring instrument, such as an attitude questionnaire, personality test or pressure sore risk calculator. These include test-retest, split-half and alternate forms. Statistical tests such as Cronbach's alpha and the Spearman rho correlation coefficient test can also be used to assess reliability.

Research method: The specific procedure used to gather and analyse research data.

Research methodology: The approach to systematic inquiry developed within a particular paradigm, with associated epistemological assumptions (e.g. experimental research, grounded theory, ethno-methodology).

Research question: A clear statement, in the form of a question, of the specific issue that a researcher wishes to answer in order to address a research problem. A research problem is an issue that lends itself to systematic investigation through research.

Response rate: The proportion (percentage) of those invited to participate in a research study who actually do so.

Retrospective study: A study that uses data about events that have already happened.

Sampling: The process of selecting a subgroup of a population to represent the entire population.

Sampling bias: The distortion that occurs when a sample is not representative of the population from which it was drawn.

Sampling error: Fluctuation in the value of a statistic from different samples drawn from the same population.

Sampling frame: A list of the entire population eligible to be included within the specific parameters of a research study. A researcher must have a sampling frame in order to generate a random sample.

Shoulder dystocia: Shoulder dystocia happens when the baby's shoulders get stuck or wedged on the mother's pubic bone after the head has been delivered. It is an obstetric emergency and the baby must be delivered as quickly as possible.

Significance level: Level of significance established at the outset by a researcher when using statistical analysis to test a hypothesis (e.g. 0.05 or 0.01). A significance level of 0.05 indicates the probability that an observed difference or relationship would be found by chance only 5 times in every 100 (1 in every 100 for a significance level of 0.01). It indicates the risk of the researcher making a type I error (i.e. an error that occurs when a researcher rejects the null hypothesis when it is true, and concludes that a statistically significant relationship/difference exists when it does not).

Statistic: A numerical datum. A numerical value, such as standard deviation or mean, that characterises the sample or population from which it was derived.

Statistical analysis: A method of analysis based on the principle of gathering data from a sample of individuals and using those data to make inferences about the wider population from which the sample was drawn.

Statistical significance: A term used to indicate whether the results of an analysis of data drawn from a sample are unlikely to have been caused by chance at a specified level of probability (usually 0.05 or 0.01).

Statistical test: A statistical procedure that allows a researcher to determine the probability that the results obtained from a sample reflect true parameters of the underlying population.

Stratified random sampling: A process which ensures that the composition of the randomly selected research group reflects the composition of the target population with respect to the stratified characteristic, e.g. age or gender.

Subjects: A term most often used in positivist research to describe those who participate in research and provide the data.

Supine: Lying on the back with the face upwards.

Survey: In the context of research, an approach that involves the systematic collection of descriptions of existing phenomena in order to describe or explain what is going on; data are obtained through direct questioning of a sample.

Syntocinon: The proprietary name of a synthetic form of the hormone oxytocin, which is sometimes given by infusion to speed up labour.

Target population: Those individuals or organisations about which one wishes to make inferences on the basis of the survey results.

Test-retest reliability: A means of assessing the stability of a research instrument by calculating the correlation between scores obtained on repeated administration.

Theme: A recurring issue that emerges during the analysis of qualitative data.

Theoretical framework: The conceptual underpinning of a research study, which may be based on theory or a specific conceptual model (in which case it may be referred to as the conceptual framework).

Theory: In its most general sense, a theory describes or explains something. Often it is the answer to a 'what', 'when', 'how' or 'why' question.

Trimester: A period of three months. The period of gestation is divided into three units of three calendar months each. Some important obstetric events may be conveniently categorised by trimesters.

Type I error: An error that occurs when a researcher rejects the null hypothesis when it is true, and concludes that a statistically significant relationship/difference exists when it does not.

Type II error: An error that occurs when a researcher accepts the null hypothesis when it is false, and concludes that no significant relationship/difference exists when it does.

Validity: In research terms, validity refers to the accuracy and truth of the data and findings produced. It applies to the concepts investigated, the people or objects studied, the methods by which the data are collected, and the findings produced. There are several different types of validity. *Face validity* is the extent to which a measuring instrument appears to those who are using it to be measuring what it claims to measure. *Internal validity* is the extent to which changes in the dependent variable (the observed effects) can be attributed to the independent variable rather than extraneous variables. *External validity* is the degree to which the results of a study are generalisable beyond the immediate study sample and setting to other samples and settings.

Variable: An attribute or characteristic of a person or object that takes on different values (i.e. it varies) within the population under investigation (e.g. age, weight, pulse rate).

Visual analogue scale: A scale used to measure clinical characteristics, such as pain or anxiety, where participants are asked to rate the characteristic on a straight line, usually with the best/worse or lowest/highest score at each extreme of the line.

References

Ackerman B (2002) Home from Home Birth Centre Statistics September 02–03. *Consultant Midwives Newsletter* **4**: 1

Active Birth Centre (1995) *Active Birth Teacher Training Prospectus.* Active Birth Centre, London

Alaily A (1996) The history of the parturition chair. In: Studd J (Ed) *The Yearbook of the Royal College of Obstetricians and Gynaecologists.* RCOG Press, London: 23-32

Aldrich CJ, D'Antona D, Spencer J et al (1995) The effect of maternal posture on fetal cerebral oxygenation during labour. *British Journal of Obstetrics and Gynaecology* **102**: 14-19

Allahbadia GN, Vaidya PR (1991) Squatting position for delivery. *Journal of the Indian Medical Association* **91**(1): 13-16

Allen CD, Ries CP (1985) Smoking, alcohol and dietary practices during pregnancy: comparison before and after prenatal education. *Journal of the American Dietetic Association* **85**(5): 605-606

Altman D (1996) Randomised trials. In: Greenfield T (Ed) *Research Methods: Guidance for Postgraduates.* John Wiley & Sons, New York: 87-94

Amos A, Jones L, Martin C (1988) *Maternity Services in Lothian: A report of a survey of user's opinions.* Maternity Services Group, Edinburgh Local Health Authority, University of Edinburgh

Anderson T, Rosser J (1998) Informed choice: was it the wrong choice? *Practising Midwife* **1**(10): 4-5

Atwood RJ (1976) Parturitional posture and related behavior. *Acta Obstetricia et Gynecologica Scandinavica. Supplement* **57**: 1-25

Audit Commission (1997) *First Class Delivery: Improving maternity care services in England and Wales.* Audit Commission, London

Audit Commission (1998) *First Class Delivery: Quality in the New NHS. A national survey of women's views of maternity care.* Belmont Press, London

Bailes A, Jackson ME (2000) Shared responsibility in home birth practice: collaborating with clients. *Journal of Midwifery and Women's Health*: **45**(6): 537-543

Ball J (1993) Workload management in midwifery In: Alexander J, Levy V, Roch S (Eds) *Midwifery Practice – A research-based approach.* Macmillan Press, Basingstoke: 154-171

Bandura A (1977) Self-efficacy: toward a unifying theory of behavioural change. *Psychological Review* **84**: 191-215

Bassell G, Humayun S, Marx G (1980) Maternal bearing down efforts – another fetal risk? *Obstetrics and Gynecology* **56**(1): 39-41

Bastian H (1994) Birth positions and the perineum: experiences and outcomes at home births in Australia. *Homebirth Australia Newsletter* **36**: 4-8

Bates R, Helm C (1985) Epidural analgesia during labour: why does this increase the forceps delivery rate? *Journal of the Royal Society of Medicine* **78**(11): 890-892

Bates R, Helm C, Duncan A, Edmonds D (1985) Uterine activity in the second stage of labour and the effect of epidural analgesia. *British Journal of Obstetrics and Gynaecology* **92**(12): 1246-1250

Beal G, Rogers E (1960) The adoption of two farm practices in a central Iowa community. Special Report 26. Agricultural and Home Economics Experiment Station, Iowa State University, Ames, Iowa. Cited in: Rogers E (1995) *Diffusion of Innovations.* The Free Press, New York: 4-19

Beasley S (2000) The value of medical publications: 'to read them would … burden the memory to no useful purpose'. *Australian and New Zealand Journal of Surgery* **70**(12): 870-874

Behnke A (2000) Expectations and the childbirth educator. *International Journal of Childbirth Education* **15**(3): 4-5

Bennett A, Hewson D, Booker E, Holliday S (1985) Antenatal preparation and labor support in relation to birth outcomes. *Birth* **12**(1): 9-16

Bevis R (1999) Obstetric anaesthesia and operations. In: Bennett R, Brown L (Eds) *Myles Textbook for Midwives.* 13th edn. Churchill Livingstone, London: 539-564

Bhardwaj N (1994) Randomised controlled trial on modified squatting position of birthing. *International Journal of Gynaecology and Obstetrics* **46**: 118

Biancuzzo M (1991) The patient observer: does the hands-and-knees posture during labour help to rotate the occiput posterior fetus? *Birth* **18**(1): 40-46

Bick D (2000a) Ask questions about practice and using appropriate methods. In: Proctor S, Renfrew M (Eds) *Linking Research and Practice in Midwifery.* Baillière Tindall, Harcourt Publications, London: 125-138

Bick D (2000b) Organisation of postnatal care and related issues. In: Alexander J, Roth C, Levy V (Eds) *Midwifery Practice – Core Topics 3.* Macmillan Press, Basingstoke: 129-142

Blaxter L, Hughes C, Tight M (1996) *How to Research.* Open University Press, Buckingham

Bodner-Adler B, Bodner K, Kimberger O, Lozanov P, Husslein P, Mayerhofer K (2003) Women's position during labour: influence on maternal and neonatal outcome. *Wiener Klinische Wochenschrift* **115**(19-20): 720-723

Bomfim-Hyppolito S (1998) Influence of the position of the mother at delivery over some maternal and neonatal outcomes. *International Journal of Gynaecology and Obstetrics* **63**(51): 67-73

Booth T (1996) Redesigning your classes to meet today's challenges. *International Journal of Childbirth Education* **May-June**, 24-25

Boyd C, Sellars L (1982) *The British Way of Birth.* Pan Books, London

Breese A (1976) Antenatal classes and preparation for pregnancy, birth and motherhood. MMedSci dissertation, Nottingham University, Nottingham

Brown S, Lumley J (1998) Communication and decision-making in labour: do birth plans make a difference? *Health Expectations* **1**(3): 106-116

Browner CH, Preloran M, Press NA (1996) The effects of ethnicity, education and an informational video on pregnant women's knowledge and decisions about a prenatal diagnostic screening test. *Patient Education and Counselling* **27**(2): 135-146

Bruner J, Drummond S, Meenan A, Gaskin I (1998) All-fours maneuver for reducing shoulder dystocia during labor. *Journal of Reproductive Medicine* **43**(5): 439-443

Burger M, Safar P (1996) Breech delivery on a delivery chair [German]. *Gynakologisch-geburtshilfliche Rundschau* **36**(2): 69-74

Burns N, Grove S (1993) *The Practice of Nursing Research*. 2nd edn. WB Saunders, Philadelphia, Pennsylvania

Byrne-Lynch A (1991) Coping strategies, personal control and childbirth. *Irish Journal of Psychology* 12(2): 145-152

Calder A, Hillan E, Stewart P (1983) A randomised study to assess the benefits and hazards of delivery in a birthing chair. MIRIAD (Midwifery Research Database) Number 0173. http://www.leeds.ac.uk (accessed 3 May 2000)

Caldeyro-Barcia R (1979a) The influence of maternal bearing down efforts during second stage on fetal well-being. *Birth and the Family Journal* 6(1): 17-21

Caldeyro-Barcia R (1979b) The influence of maternal position on time of spontaneous rupture of the membranes, progress of labor and fetal head compression. *Birth and the Family Journal* 6(1): 7-15

Campbell R, MacFarlane A (1986) Place of delivery: a review. *British Journal of Obstetrics and Gynaecology* 93(7): 675-683

Campbell R, MacFarlane A (1990) Recent debate on the place of birth. In: Garcia J, Kilpatrick F, Richards M (Eds) *The Politics of Maternity Care*. Oxford University Press, Oxford: 217-237

Carlson JM, Diehl JA, Sachtleben-Murray M, McRae M, Fenwick L, Friedman EA (1986) Maternal position during parturition in normal labor. *Obstetrics and Gynecology* 68(4): 443-447

Cartwright A (1979) *The Dignity of Labour: A study of childbearing and induction*. Tavistock, London

Chamberlain G (2000) Choosing between home and hospital delivery: risk of home birth in Britian cannot be compared with data from other countries. *British Medical Journal* 320(3): 798

Chan D (1963) Positions during labour. *British Medical Journal* i(5323): 100-102

Chen SZ, Aisaka K, Mori H, Kigawa T (1987) Effects of sitting position on uterine activity during labor. *Obstetrics and Gynecology* 69(1): 67-73

Churchill H, Benbow A (2000) Informed choice in maternity services. *British Journal of Midwifery* 8(1): 41-47

Clancy C, Cebul R, Williams S (1988) Guiding individual decisions: a randomized, controlled trial of decision analysis. *American Journal of Medicine* 84(2): 283-288

Clark E (2000) The historical context of research in midwifery. In: Proctor S, Renfrew M (Eds) *Linking Research and Practice in Midwifery: A guide to evidence-based practice*. Baillière Tindall, Edinburgh: 35-54

Clements R (1994) An investigation of the extent to which the demand for, and uptake of, alternative birth positions by mothers in a teaching hospital is led by the midwife. BSc(Health) dissertation, Leeds College of Health, University of Leeds

Cliff D, Deery R (1997) Too much like school: social class, age, marital status and attendance/ non-attendance at antenatal classes. *Midwifery* 13(3): 139-145

Clifford J, Marcus G (1986) *Writing Culture – The poetics and politics of ethnography*. University of California Press, Berkeley

Cluett E (2000) An introduction to statistics in midwifery research. In: Cluett E, Bluff R (Eds) *Principles and Practice of Research in Midwifery*. Baillière Tindall, Edinburgh: 79-112

Cluett E, Bluff R (2000) From practice to research. In: Cluett E, Bluff R (Eds) *Principles and Practice of Research in Midwifery*. Baillière Tindall, Edinburgh: 11-26

Coffin A (1995) *Treatise on Midwifery and the Diseases of Women and Children*. 13th edn. Yesterday's Books, Berkshire

Combes G, Schonveld A (1992) *Life Will Never be the Same Again*. Health Education Authority, London

COMET (Comparative Obstetric Mobile Epidural Trial) Study Group UK (2001) Effect of low-dose mobile versus traditional epidural techniques on mode of delivery: a randomised controlled trial. *Lancet* 358(9275):19-23

Coppen R (1994) Consumer views of maternity care in Mid-Surrey. In: *MIRIAD*. 1st edn. Books for Midwives Press, Cheshire

Coppen R (1997) Midwives' views on the use of alternative positions in their place of practice. Research presented during a Midwives' Study Day Workshop, July, Kings College London University, London

Coppen R (1999) A comparative survey of midwives' knowledge and preference of birthing positions in two countries and three settings: Thomson Medical Centre, Kandang Kerbau Hospital (Singapore) and Epsom General Hospital (UK). Seminar presentation, July 2002, Singapore

Coppen R (2002) Collaborating with women on their choice of birthing positions: a decision making approach to apply focused information as a strategy to enhance knowledge and reduce decision conflict in pregnancy and childbirth. PhD thesis, UniS Library/Archives, University of Surrey, UK

Copstick S, Hayes R, Taylor K, Morris N (1985) A test of common assumptions regarding the use of antenatal training during labour. *Journal of Psychosomatic Research* **29**: 215-218

Cottrell B, Shannahan M (1986) Effect of the birth chair on duration of second stage labour and maternal outcome. *Nursing Research* **35**(6): 364-367

Cottrell B, Shannahan M (1987) A comparison of fetal outcome in birth chair and delivery table births. *Research in Nursing and Health* **10**: 239-243

Cronbach L (1990) *Essentials of Psychological Testing*. 5th edn. Harper Row, New York

Crowley P, Elbourne D, Ashurst H, Garcia J, Murphy D, Duignan N (1991) Delivery in an obstetric birth chair: a randomised controlled trial. *British Journal of Obstetrics and Gynaecology* **198**: 667-674

Currell R (1990) The organisation of midwifery care. In: Alexander J, Levy V, Roch S (Eds) *Midwifery Practice – Antenatal Care: A research-based approach*. MacMillan Press, London

Davis C (2002) Change fatigue. *NursingTimes* **98**(2): 23-24

De Jong P, Johanson R, Baxen P, Adrians V, van der Westhuisen S, Jones P (1997) Randomised trial comparing the upright and supine positions for the second stage of labour. *British Journal of Obstetrics and Gynaecology* **104**(5): 567-571

De Jonge A, Lagro-Janssen A (2004) Birthing positions: a qualitative study into the views of women about various birthing positions. *Journal of Psychosomatic Obstetrics and Gynaecology* **25**(1): 47-55

De Jonge A, Teunissen T, Lagro-Nahssen A (2004) Supine position compared to other positions during the second stage of labor: a meta-analytic review. *Journal of Psychosomatic Obstetrics and Gynaecology* **25**(1): 35-45

De Lee J (1934) Obstetrics versus midwifery. *Journal of the American Medical Association* **103**: 307

Dening F (1982) The woman's stool or the parturition chair. *Midwives Chronicle and Nursing Notes* **95**(1): 440-442

Department of Health (1993) *Changing Childbirth Part I: Report of the Expert Maternity Group* (Cumberlege Report). HMSO, London

Department of Health (1997) *The New NHS: Modern, dependable*. The Stationery Office, London

Department of Health (1998a) *Recruitment and Retention Campaign*. Department of Health, London: 1-2

Department of Health (1998b) *A First Class Service: Quality in the new NHS*. The Stationery Office, London

Department of Health (2000) *Department of Health Working Lives: Programmes for change*. Department of Health Recruitment and Retention Unit, London

Department of Health (2001) *Campaign to Bring Midwives Back to the NHS*. Department of Health, London: 1

Department of Health (2004) *National Service Framework for Children, Young People and Maternity Care.* DH, UK. Also www.dh.gov.uk (accessed 22.6.05)

Department of Health (2005) *Evidence to Inform the National Service Framework for Children, Young People and Maternity Services.* DH, UK. Also gateway reference 2005: www.dh.gov.uk (accessed 22.6.05)

Diaz A, Schwarcz R, Fescina R, Caldeyro-Barcia R (1980) Vertical position during the first stage of the course of labor, and neonatal outcome. *European Journal of Obstetrics, Gynecology and Reproductive Biology* **11**(1): 1-7

Diepgen P (1937) Cited in: Housholder M (1974) A historical perspective on the obstetric chair. *Surgery, Gynecology and Obstetrics* **139**: 424

Dimond B (1997) CESDI 2: The legal implications. *Modern Midwife* **7**(12): 20-22

Dimond B (2001) Litigation in the NHS: Recommendations for change. *British Journal of Midwifery* **9**(7): 443-446

Dingwall R (1993) Negligence and litigation research and the practice of midwifery. In: Alexander J, Levy V, Roch S (Eds) *Midwifery Practice – A research-based approach.* MacMillan Press, London

Dobson F (1998) Foreword by the Secretary of State. In: Department of Health (1998) *A First Class Service: Quality in the New NHS.* http://www.open.gov.uk/newnhs/ quality.htm (accessed 20 June 2000)

Dodwell M, Armes R (2001) www.BirthChoiceUK.com. *British Journal of Midwifery* **9**(7): 425

Dolan J (1999) A method for evaluating health care providers' decision-making: The provider decision process instrument. *Medical Decision-Making* **19**(1): 38-41

Donovan P (2000) Ethnography. In: Cluett E, Bluff R (Eds) *Principles and Practice of Research in Midwifery.* Baillière Tindall, Harcourt Publishing, Edinburgh: 131-148

Downe S, Gerrett D, Renfrew M (2004) A prospective randomised trial on the effect of position in the passive second stage of labour on birth outcome in nulliparous women using epidural analgesia. *Midwifery* **20**(2): 157-168

Dundes L (1987) The evolution of maternal birthing position. *American Journal of Public Health* **77**(5): 636–641

Dunn P (1991) François Mauriceau (1637–1709) and maternal posture for parturition. *Archives of Disease in Childhood* **669**(1 Spec No): 78–79

Eastwood R (1940) *Sales Control of Quantitative Methods.* Columbia, USA

Eiser JR (1998) Communication and interpretation of risk. *British Medical Bulletin* **54**(4): 779-790

Englemann G (1882) *Labor Among Primitive Peoples.* St Louis, JH Chambers: 66-73

Enkin M, Keirse M, Neilson J et al (2000) *A Guide to Effective Care in Pregnancy and Childbirth.* 3rd edn. Oxford University Press, Oxford

Estabrooks C, Goel V, Thiel E, Pinfold P, Sawka C, Williams I (2001) Decision aids: are they worth it? A systematic review. *Journal of Health Services and Research Policy* **6**(3):170-182

Fasbender H (1906) Geschichte der Gerburtshülfe, p 156, Jena, Gustav Fischer, Germany. Cited in: Shorter E (1991) A typical birth then. In: *Women's Bodies – A social history of women's encounter with health, ill health and medicine.* Transaction Publishers, New Jersey, USA: 48-68

Fenwick L, Simkin P (1987) Maternal positioning to prevent or alleviate dystocia in labor. *Clinical Obstetrics and Gynecology* **30**(1): 83-90

Fields H, Greene J, Smith K (1965) *Induction of Labour.* Macmillan, New York

Fischhoff B, Beyth-Marom R (1988) Clinical decision analysis. In: Dowie J, Elstein A (Eds) (1988) *Professional Judgement: A reader in clinical decision-making.* Cambridge University Press, Cambridge: 409-424

Fletcher RH, Fletcher SW (1998) The future of medical journals in the Western world. *Lancet* **175**: 30-33

Ford S (1945) *A Comparative Study of Human Reproduction.* Yale University Publication in Anthropology, No. 32. Yale University Press, New Haven, Connecticut

Foster Dr (2001) The Good Birth Guide. *Sunday Times Magazine Supplement.* 15 July 2001. The Sunday Times Press, UK

Foster Dr (2005) The Good Birth Guide. www.drfoster.co.uk (accessed 22 May 2005)

Gagnon A (2001) Individual or group antenatal education for childbirth/parenthood (Cochrane Review). In: *The Cochrane Library* 2001 (3): CD002869. John Wiley & Sons, Chichester

Gallo C, Perrone F, De Placido S, Giusti C (1995) Informed versus randomised consent to clinical trials. *Lancet* **364** (8982): 1060-1064

Garcia J (1982) Women's views of antenatal care. In: Enkin M, Chalmers I (Eds) *Effectiveness and Satisfaction in Antenatal Care.* Heinemann Medical, London

Garcia J, Garforth S, Ayers S (1986) Midwives confined: labour ward policies and routines. *Research and the Midwife Conference Proceedings,* University of Manchester: 74-80

Garcia J, Kilpatrick R, Richards M (Eds])(1990) *The Politics Of Maternity Care: Services for childbearing women in twentieth century Britain.* Clarendon Press, Oxford.

Gardosi J, Sylvester S, B-Lynch C (1989a) Alternative positions in the second stage of labour: a randomized controlled trial. *British Journal of Obstetrics and Gynaecology* **96**(11): 1290-1296

Gardosi J, Hutson N, B-Lynch C (1989b) Randomised controlled trial of squatting in the second stage of labour. *Lancet* **2**(8654): 74-79

Garrison P (1929) *An Introduction to the History of Medicine.* 4th edn. WB Saunders, Philadelphia: 277

Garrud P, Wood M, Standsby L (2001) Impact of risk information in a patient education leaflet. *Patient Education and Counseling* **43**(3):301-304

Glaser B (1992) *Basics of Grounded Theory Analysis.* Sociology Press, Mill Valley, California

Goer H (1999) *The Thinking Woman's Guide to a Better Birth.* Berkeley Publishing Group, Berkley

Golay J, Vedam S, Sorger L (1993) The squatting positions for the 2nd stage of labour: effects on labour and on maternal and fetal well-being. *Birth* **20**(2): 73-78

Goodfellow C, Hull M, Swaab D, Dogterom J, Buijs R (1983) Oxytocin deficiency at delivery with epidural analgesia. *British Journal of Obstetrics and Gynaecology* **90**(3): 214-219

Goodwin L (1997) Changing conceptions of measurement validity. *Journal of Nurse Education* **36**(3):102-107

Government Statistical Service for the Department of Health (2005) *NHS Maternity Statistics, England: 2003-04.* Statistical Bulletin 2005/10

Graham H (1984) *Women, Health and the Family.* Wheatsheaf Books, Brighton

Graham H (1960) *Eternal Eve: The mysteries of birth and the customs that surround it.* Hutchinson, London

Gray J (1997) *Evidence-Based Healthcare.* Churchill Livingstone, Edinburgh

Green J (1993) Expectations and experiences of pain in labour: findings from a large prospective study. *Birth* **20**: 65-72

Green J, Coupland V, Kitzinger J (1990a) Expectations, experiences and psychological outcomes of childbirth: a prospective study of 825 women. *Birth* **17**(1): 15-24

Green J, Kitzinger J, Coupland V (1990b) Stereotypes of childbearing women: a look at some evidence. *Midwifery* **6**(3): 125-132

Greenfield T (1996) Laboratory and industrial experiments. In: Greenfield T (Ed) *Research Methods: Guidance for Postgraduates.* Arnold, London: 97-106

Gupta J, Hofmeyr G (2004) Position for women during second stage of labour (Cochrane Review). In: *The Cochrane Library* 2004 (1): CD002006. John Wiley & Sons, Chichester

Gupta J, Lilford R (1987) Birth positions. *Midwifery* **3**: 92-96

Gupta J, Nikodem V (2000a) Woman's position during second stage of labour (Cochrane

Review). In: *The Cochrane Library* 2000 (2): CD002006. John Wiley & Sons, Chichester

Gupta J, Nikodem V (2000b) Maternal posture in labour. *European Journal of Obstetrics, Gynecology and Reproductive Biology* **92**(2): 273-277

Gupta J, Brayshaw E, Lilford R (1989a) An experiment of squatting birth. *European Journal of Obstetrics, Gynecology and Reproductive Biology* **30**(3): 217-220

Gupta J, Leal C, Johnson N, Lilford R (1989b) Squatting in second stage of labour. *Lancet* **2**(8662): 561-562

Haidet P, Hamel M, Davis S et al (1998) Outcomes, preferences for resuscitation, and physician-patient communication among patients with metastatic colorectal cancer. SUPPORT Investigators. Study to Understand Prognoses and Preferences for Outcomes and Risks of Treatments. *American Journal of Medicine* **105**(3): 222-229

Hallgren A, Kihlgren M, Norberg A, Forslin L (1995) Women's perceptions of childbirth and childbirth education before and after education and birth. *Midwifery* **11**(3): 130-137

Handfield B (1997) The trouble with childbirth education. *Birth Issues* **6**(1): 5-7

Hanson L (1998a) Second stage positioning in nurse-midwifery practices. Part 1: Position use and preferences. *Journal of Nurse-Midwifery* **43**(5): 320-325

Hanson L (1998b) Second stage positioning in nurse-midwifery practices. Part 2: Factors affecting use. *Journal of Nurse-Midwifery* **43**(5): 326–330

Hemminki E, Virkunnen A, Makela A et al (1986) A trial of delivery in a birth chair. *Journal of Obstetrics and Gynaecology* **6**(3): 162-165

Henty D (1998) Brought to bed: a critical look at birthing positions. *Midwives* **1**(10): 310-313

Hetherington S (1990) A controlled study of the effect of prepared childbirth classes on obstetric outcomes. *Birth* **17**(2): 86-90

Hewes G (1957) The anthropology of posture. *Scientific American* **96**: 122-132

Hibbard B, Robinson J, Pearson J, Rosen M, Taylor A (1979) The effectiveness of antenatal education. *Health Education Journal* **38**(2): 39-46

Higgins R (1996) *Approaches to Research*. Jessica Kingsley Publishers, London

Hillan E (1996) Caesarean section in conception, pregnancy and birth. In: Niven C, Walker A (Eds) *Conception, Pregnancy and Birth*. Butterworth-Heinemann, Oxford: 120-130

Hillier D (2003) *Childbirth in the Global Village: Implications for midwifery education and practice*. Routledge, London

Hillier C, Slade P (1989) The impact of antenatal classes on knowledge, anxiety and confidence in primiparous women. *Journal of Reproductive and Infant Psychology* **7**: 3-13

Hoddinott P, Pill R (1999) Nobody actually tells you: a study of infant feeding. *British Journal of Midwifery* **7**(9): 558-565

Holloway I, Wheeler S (1996a) Grounded theory. In: *Qualitative Research for Nurses*. Blackwell Science, Oxford: 98-114

Holloway I, Wheeler S (1996b) *Qualitative Research for Nurses*. Blackwell Science, Oxford

Horey D, Weaver J, Russell H (2004) Information for pregnant women about caesarean birth (Cochrane Review). In: *The Cochrane Library* 2004 (1): CD003858. John Wiley & Sons, Chichester

House of Commons Health Select Committee (1992) *Second Report on the Maternity Services* (Winterton Report). HMSO, London

Housham K (1998) How informed are pregnant women about their choice of delivery positions in the antenatal period? Unpublished BSc(Hons) Midwifery dissertation, King's College, London

Housholder M (1974) A historical perspective on the obstetric chair. *Surgery, Gynecology and Obstetrics* **139**: 423-430

Howard F (1958) Delivery in the physiologic position. *Obstetrics and Gynecology* **11**(3): 318-322

Howell C (2000) Epidural versus non-epidural analgesia for pain relief in labour (Cochrane Review). In: *The Cochrane Library* 2000 (2): CD000331. John Wiley & Sons, Chichester

Howell C (2004) Epidural versus non-epidural analgesia for pain relief in labour (Cochrane Review). In: *The Cochrane Library* 2004 (3): CD000331. John Wiley & Sons, Chichester

Humphrey M, Hounslow D, Morgan S, Wood D (1973) The influence of maternal posture at birth on the fetus. *The Journal of Obstetrics and Gynaecology of the British Commonwealth* **80**(12): 1075–1080

Hundley V, Milne J, Leyton-Beck L, Graham W, Fitzmaurice A (2000) Raising research awareness among midwives and nurses: does it work? *Journal of Advanced Nursing* **31**(1): 78-88

Husband L (1983) Antenatal education: its use and effectiveness. *Health Visitor* **56**: 409-410

Hutchinson A (1986) Grounded theory: the method. In: Munhall P, Oiler C (Eds) *Nursing Research: A qualitative perspective*. Appleton-Century-Croft, Newark, Connecticut

Inch S (1982a) The assumption of pathology and its implications. In: *Birthrights – A parent's guide to modern childbirth* . Hutchinson & Co, London: 26-42

Inch S (1982b) The second stage. In: *Birthrights – A parent's guide to modern childbirth*. Hutchinson & Co, London: 117-144

Ivey S, Brown K, Teske Y, Silverman D (1988) A model for teaching about interdisciplinary practice in health care settings. *Journal of Allied Health* **17**(3): 189-195

Izzo J (1994) Partnership, not empowerment, creates excellent organizations. *Managed Care Quarterly* **2**(1): 50-53

Jacoby A (1998) Mothers' views about information and advice in pregnancy and childbirth: findings from a national study. *Midwifery* **4**(3): 103-110

Jadad A (1998) *Randomised Controlled Trials*. BMJ Publishing Group, London

Jamieson L (1994) Midwife empowerment through education. *British Journal of Midwifery* **12**(2): 47-48

Jansen P, Blizzard S (1999) Childbirth education: does it meet women's needs? *Current Practice Perspectives Open Line* **7**(4): 1, 10-11

Jarcho J (1929) The role of posture in obstetrics. *Surgery, Gynecology and Obstetrics* **48**: 257-264

Jarcho J (1934) *Posture and Practices during Labour among Primitive Peoples*. Hoeber, New York

Johnstone F, Aboelmagd M, Harouny A (1987) Maternal posture in second stage and fetal acid base status. *British Journal of Obstetrics and Gynaecology* **94**(8): 753-757

Jordan B (1993) *Birth in Four Cultures: A cross-cultural investigation of childbirth in Yucatan, Holland, Sweden and the United States*. 4th edn. Prospect Heights, Waveland Press, Illinois, US

Jordan B (1997) Authoritative knowledge and its construction. In: Davis-Floyd R, Sargent C (Eds) *Childbirth and Authoritative Knowledge: Cross-cultural perspectives*. University of California Press, California

Jordan B, Irwin S (1989) The ultimate failure – court ordered caesarean section. Cited in: Sargent C, Bascope G (1996) Ways of knowing about birthing in three cultures. *Medical Anthropology Quarterly* **10**(2): 213-236

Kafka M, Riss P, von Trotsenburg M (1994) The birthing stool – an obstetrical risk? (German) *Geburtshilfe Frauenheilkd* **54**(9): 529–531

Kaufert P, O'Neil J (1993) Analysis of a dialogue on risks in childbirth clinicians – clinicians, epidemiologists and Inuit women. In: Lindenbaum S, Lock M (Eds) *Knowledge, Power and Practice – The anthropology of medicine and everyday life*. University of California Press, Berkeley: 32-55

Keleher K (1998) Collaborative practice: characteristics, barriers, benefits and implications for midwifery. *Journal of Nurse-Midwifery* **43**(1): 8-11

Kelly B, Sandall J, Fitzgerald L, Harvey J (2001) Delivering maternity care: does control in childbirth matter to women? Poster presentation at the Research in Midwifery Conference, Birmingham, 3 April 2001

Kelly F, Terry R, Naglieri R (1999) A review of the alternative birthing positions. *Journal of the American Obstetrics Association (JAOA)* **99**(9): 470–474

Kirkham M (1989) Midwives and information giving during labour. In: Robinson S, Thomson A (Eds) *Midwives, Research and Childbirth, Volume 1*. Chapman and Hall, London: 117-138

Kirkham M (1993) Communication in midwifery. In: Alexander J, Levy V, Roch S (Eds) *Midwifery Practice – A research-based approach*. Macmillan, Basingstoke: 1-19

Kitzinger S (1983) *The New Good Birth Guide*. Penguin Books, Harmondsworth, Middlesex

Kitzinger S (1988) *Some Women's Experiences of Epidurals*. National Childbirth Trust, London

Kitzinger S (1999) Birth plans: how are they being used? *British Journal of Midwifery* 7(5): 300-303

Kitzinger S, Davis J (1978) *The Place of Birth*. Oxford University Press, Oxford

Kitzinger S, Walters R (1981) *Some Women's Experiences of Episiotomy*. National Childbirth Trust, London

Kleine-Tebbe A, David M, Farkic D (1996) Upright birthing position – more birth canal injuries? Results of a retrospective comparative study (German). *Zentralblatt fur Gynakologie* 118(18): 448-452

Kloosterman G (1975) The assumption of pathology. In: Inch S (Ed) *Birthrights*. Hutchinson and Co., London: 26-42

Knauth D, Haloburdo E (1986) Effect of pushing techniques in birthing chair on length of second stage of labour. *Nursing Research* 35(1): 49-51

Larson M (1997) Alternative delivery position and perineal integrity for primigravidae. Unpublished MSc dissertation, University of Surrey/Royal College of Midwives, Surrey

Lauzon L, Hodnett E (1998) Antenatal education for self-diagnosis of the onset of active labour at term. In: *The Cochrane Library* 1998 (3): CD000935. John Wiley & Sons, Chichester

Lavender T, Walkinshaw S, Walton I (1999) A prospective study of women's views of factors contributing to a positive birth experience. *Midwifery* 15(1): 40-46

Lee H, Shorten A (1999) Childbirth education: do classes meet consumer expectations? *Birth Issues* 7(4): 137-142

Leishman W (1879) *A System of Midwifery, including the Diseases of Pregnancy and the Puerperal State*. 3rd edn. Henry C Lea, Philadelphia

Levy V (1999a) Midwives, informed choice and power: Part 1. *British Journal of Midwifery* 7(9): 583-586

Levy V (1999b) Midwives, informed choice and power: Part 2. *British Journal of Midwifery* 7(10): 613-616

Levy V (1999c) Midwives, informed choice and power: Part 3. *British Journal of Midwifery* 7(11): 694-699

Levy V (1999d) Maintaining equilibrium: a grounded theory study of the processes involved when women make informed choices during pregnancy. *Midwifery* 15(2):109-19

Lewis J (1990) Mothers and maternity policies in the twentieth century. In: Garcia J, Kilpatrick R, Richards M (Eds) *The Politics of Maternity Care*. Clarendon Press, Oxford: 15-29

Ley P (1982a) Satisfaction, compliance and communication. *British Journal of Clinical Psychology* 21: 241-254

Ley P (1982b) Giving information to patients. In: Eise J (Ed) *Social Psychology and Behavioural Medicine*. John Wiley & Sons, Chichester

Ley P (1988) *Communicating with Patients*. Psychology and Medicine Series. Croom Helm, London

Libbus M, Sable M (1991) Prenatal education in a high-risk population: the effect on birth outcomes. *Birth* 18(2): 78-82

Liddell H, Fisher P (1985) The birthing chair in the second stage of labour. *The Australian & New Zealand Journal of Obstetrics and Gynaecology* 25(1): 65-68

Lilford R, Pauker S, Braunholtz D, Chard J (1998) Decision analysis and the implementation of research findings. *British Medical Journal* 317(7155): 405-409

Limburg A, Smulders B (1992) *Women Giving Birth: Vertical Delivery*. Celestial Arts, Berkeley, California

Lindenbaum S, Lock M (Eds) (1993) *Knowledge, Power and Practice – The anthropology of medicine and everyday life.* University of California Press, Berkeley

Litt M (1988) Self-efficacy and perceived control: cognitive mediators of pain tolerance. *Journal of Personality and Social Psychology* **54**(1):149-160

Liu E, Sia A (2004) Rates of caesarean section and instrumental vaginal delivery in nulliparous women after low concentration epidural infusions or opioid analgesia: systematic review. *British Medical Journal* **328**(7453): 1410

Liu YC (1986) Effect of an upright position during childbirth. In: *Proceedings of the 1st National Research Conference on Living with Change and Choice in Health.* University of West Virginia, West Virginia, USA

Liu YC (1988) The effects of the upright position during childbirth. *Journal of Nursing Scholarship* **8 September**: 14-18

Logue M (1991) Putting research into practice: perineal management during delivery. In: Robinson S, Thomson A (Eds) *Midwives, Research and Childbirth, Volume 2.* Chapman and Hall, London: 252-270

Lumley J, Brown S (1993) Attenders and non-attenders at childbirth education classes in Australia: how do they and their births differ? *Birth* **20**(3): 123-130

Lusk W (1894) *The Science and Art of Midwifery.* D Appleton & Co., New York

MacFarlane A, Mugford M (1984) *Birth Counts: Statistics of pregnancy and childbirth.* HMSO, London

Machin D, Scamell A (1998) Using ethnographic research to examine effects of 'informed choice'. *British Journal of Midwifery* **6**(5): 304-309

MacLennan A (1978) An audit of obsolete practice in the management of labour. *The Australian & New Zealand Journal of Obstetrics and Gynaecology* **18**: 287-288

MacLeod-Clark J (1985) The development of research. In: Kagan C (Ed) *Interpersonal Skills in Nursing.* Croom Helm, London

Marcus G, Fischer M (1986) *Anthropology as Cultural Critique: An experimental moment in the human sciences.* University of Chicago Press, Chicago

Madi B (2000) Women's decision-making and factors affecting their choice of place of delivery. Unpublished PhD thesis, EIHMS, University of Surrey

Mander R (1993) Who chooses the choices? *Modern Midwife* **3**: 23-25

Maresh M, Choong KH, Beard R (1983) Delayed pushing with lumbar epidural analgesia in labour. *British Journal of Obstetrics and Gynaecology* **90**(7): 623-627

Martilla M, Kajanoja P, Ylikorkala O (1983) Maternal half-sitting position in the second stage of labour. *Journal of Perinatal Medicine* **11**: 286-289

Martin A (1917) Cited in: Shorter E (1991) A typical birth then – a history of the birth experience. In: *Women's Bodies – A Social History of Women's Encounter with Health, Ill Health and Medicine.* Transaction Publishers, New Jersey, USA: 48-68

Mason V (1989) *Women's Experiences of Maternity Care – A survey manual.* HMSO, London

Maternity Care Working Party (2000) *The Case for a National Service Framework for Maternity Care.* Maternity Care Working Party, London: 1-2

Maternity Services Advisory Committee (1982) *Maternity Care in Action: Part 1 – Antenatal Care.* HMSO, Basildon

Maternity Services Advisory Committee (1984) *Maternity Care in Action: Part II – Care During Childbirth.* HMSO, Basildon

Maternity Services Advisory Committee (1985) *Maternity Care in Action Part III – Care of the Mother and the Baby.* HMSO, Basildon

Mayer K (1942) Uber den Gebarstühl, p7-1, Erlangen: Junge & Sohn. Cited in Housholder M (1974) A historical perspective on the obstetric chair. *Surgery, Gynecology and Obstetrics* **139**: 424

McCabe F, Rocheron Y, Dickson R, McCron R (1984) *Antenatal Education in Primary Care: A survey of general practitioners, midwives and health visitors.* Centre for Mass Communication Research, University of Leicester, Leicester

McGuire W (1989) Theoretical foundation of campaigns. In: Rice R, Atkins C (Eds) *Public Communication Campaigns.* 2nd edn. Sage, Newbury Park, CA: 43-65

McIntosh J (1988) A consumer view of birth preparation classes: attitudes of a sample of working class primigravidae. *Midwives' Chronicle* **101**(1199): 8-9

McKay S (1980) Maternal position during labor and birth: a reassessment. *Journal of Obstetric, Gynecologic and Neonatal Nursing* **9**(5): 288–291

McKay S (1984) Squatting: an alternate position for the second stage of labor. *The American Journal of Maternal Child Nursing* **9**(3): 181-183

McKay S, Mahan C (1984) Laboring patients need more freedom to move. *Contemporary Obstetrics and Gynecology*, **July**: 90-119

McLain B (1988) Collaborative practice: a critical theory perspective. *Research in Nursing and Health* **11**: 391-398

McManus T, Calder A (1978) Upright posture and the efficiency of labour. *Lancet* **1**(8055): 72-74

McQueen J, Mylrea L (1977) Lumbar epidural analgesia in labour. *British Medical Journal* **1**: 640-641

Michie S, Marteau T, Kidd J (1992) Predicting antenatal class attendance: attitudes of self and others. *Psychology and Health* 7: 225-234

MIDIRS (1996) *Positions in Labour* and *Delivery: Informed Choice for Women and Professionals* (Leaflets). MIDIRS and The NHS Centre for Reviews and Dissemination, London

MIDIRS (2003) *Positions in Labour* and *Delivery: Informed Choice for Women and Professionals* (Leaflets). MIDIRS and The NHS Centre for Reviews and Dissemination, Plus One Design, Bristol

Miller D (1991) *Handbook of Research Design and Social Measurement.* 5th edn. Sage Publications, London

Molenaar S, Sprangers M, Postma-Schuit F et al (2000) Feasibility and effects of decision aids. *Medical Decision-Making* **20**(1): 112-127

Moore S (1997) Psychosocial support during labour. In: Henderson C, Jones K (Eds) *Essential Midwifery.* Mosby, London: 219-227

Moser C, Katton G (1971) *Survey Methods in Social Investigation.* 2nd edn. Heinemann, London

Murphy-Black T (1990) Antenatal education. In: Alexander J, Levy V, Roch S (Eds) *Antenatal Care: A research-based approach.* Macmillan Education, Basingstoke: 88-104

Murphy-Black T (1991) Antenatal education: evaluation of post-basic training course. In: Robinson S, Thomson A (Eds) *Midwives, Research and Childbirth. Volume I.* Chapman and Hall, London

Naroll F, Naroll R, Howard F (1961) Position of women in childbirth: a study in data quality control. *American Journal of Obstetrics and Gynecology* **82**: 943-954

National Childbirth Trust (1991) NCT Teachers' Annual Returns (1990) *Outreach.* NCT, London

National Childbirth Trust (1995) *Birth Choices: Women's Expectations and Experiences.* NCT, London

National Institute for Clinical Excellence (NICE) (2003) *Antenatal Care. Clinical Guideline 5.* National Collaborating Centre for Women's & Children's Health and NICE, London

Nelki J, Bond L (1995) Positions in labour: a plea for flexibility. *Modern Midwife* **5**(2):19-22

New King James Bible (2000) Exodus 1:16. New King James Version, Nelson Bibles, US

Newburn M (2000) Informed choice – are we getting there? *RCM Midwives Journal* **3**(9): 278-281

Newton N (1957) The effect of position on the course of the second stage of labor. *Surgical Forum* **7**: 517-520

Newton ER, Schroeder BC, Knape KG, Bennett BL (1995) Epidural analgesia and uterine function.

Obstetrics and Gynecology **85**(5 Pt 1): 749-755

NHS Centre for Reviews and Dissemination (1996) *NHS Centre for Reviews and Dissemination.* York Publishing Services, University of York, UK

NHS Centre for Reviews and Dissemination (2001) *Undertaking Systematic Reviews of Research on Effectiveness.* CRD Report No. 4 (2nd edn). http://www.york.ac.uk (accessed June 2001)

Nichols F, Humerick S (1988) *Childbirth Education: Practice, Research and Theory.* WB Saunders Company, Philadelphia, PA.

Nichols M (1993) Adjustment to new parenthood: attenders versus non-attenders at prenatal education classes. *Birth* **2**(1): 21-26

Nikodem V (1995) Upright vs recumbent position during second stage of labour (Pre-Cochrane Review). In: *The Cochrane Library* 2000 (2): CD. John Wiley & Sons, Chichester

Niven C (1986) Factors affecting labour pain. Doctoral thesis, University of Stirling, Scotland

Niven C (1992) *Psychological Care for Families Before, During and After Birth.* Butterworth-Heinemann, Oxford

Niven C, Gijsbers K (1996) Perinatal pain. In: Niven C, Walker A (Eds) *Conception, Pregnancy and Birth.* Butterworth-Heinemann, Oxford: 131-147

Nodine P, Roberts J (1987) Factors associated with perineal outcome during childbirth. *Journal of Nurse-Midwifery* **32**(3): 123-130

Nolan M (1995) A comparison of attenders at antenatal classes in the voluntary and statutory sectors: education and organisational implications. *Midwifery* **11**(3): 138-145

Nolan M (1997) Antenatal education – where next? *Journal of Advanced Nursing* **25**(6): 1198-1204

Nolan M (1998) *Antenatal Education: A dynamic approach.* Baillière Tindall, London

Nolan M (1999) Antenatal education: past and future agendas. *Practising Midwife* **2**(3): 24-27

Nolan M, Hicks C (1997) Aims, processes and problems of antenatal education as identified by three groups of childbirth teachers. *Midwifery* **13**(4): 179-188

Nunnally D, Aguiar M (1974) Patients' evaluation of their prenatal and delivery care. *Nursing Research* **23**(6): 469-474

Oakley A (1980) *Women Confined: Towards a sociology of childbirth.* Martin Robertson and Company, Oxford

Oakley A (1986) *The Captured Womb: A history of the medical care of pregnant women.* 2nd edn. Basil Blackwell, Oxford

Oakley A, Richard M (1990) Women's experience of caesarean delivery. In: Garcia J, Kilpatrick, Richards M (Eds) *The Politics of Maternity Care: Services for childbearing women in twentieth century Britain.* Clarendon Press, Oxford: 183-201

O'Cathain A, Thomas K, Walters SJ, Nicholl J, Kirkham M (2002) Women's perceptions of informed choice in maternity care. *Midwifery* **18**(2): 136-44

O'Connor A (1995) Validation of a decisional conflict scale. *Medical Decision-Making* **15**(1): 25-29

O'Connor A, Rostom A, Fiset V et al (1999) Decision aids for patients facing health treatment or screening decisions: systematic review. *British Medical Journal* **319**(7212): 731-734

O'Connor AM, Stacey D, Entwistle V et al (2003) Decision aids for people facing health treatment or screening decisions. In: *The Cochrane Library* 2003 (1): CD001431. John Wiley & Sons, Chichester

Odent M (1984) *Birth Reborn.* Souvenir Press, London

Oliver S, Rajan L, Turner H et al (1996) A pilot study of 'Informed choice' leaflets on positions in labour and routine ultrasound. The University of York NHS Centre for Reviews and Dissemination, CRD Report No. 7: 1-47. http://www.york.ac.uk. (accessed 1 November 1999)

Oppenheim A (1992) *Questionnaire Design, Interviewing and Attitude Measurement.* 2nd edn. Pinter, London

Oxford English Dictionary (2000) *Oxford (Compact) English Dictionary.* Completely New Edition. Oxford University Press, Oxford

Paciornik M (1990) Arguments against episiotomy and in favour of squatting for birth. *Birth* **17**(2): 104-105

Parahoo A (1997) *Nursing Research – Principles, process and issues.* Macmillan, Basingstoke

Peat J (2002) *Health Science Research – A handbook of qualitative methods.* Sage Publications, London

Pocock S (1992) When to stop a clinical trial. *British Medical Journal* **305**(6847): 235-240

Polit D, Beck C (2003) *Nursing Research: Principles and methods.* 7th edn. JB Lippincott Co., Philadelphia, US

Polit D, Hungler B (1983) *Nursing Research: Principles and methods.* 2nd edn. JB Lippincott Co., Philadelphia, US

Polit D, Hungler B (1997) *Essentials of Nursing Research: Methods, appraisal, and utilization.* 4th edn. Lippincott Williams & Wilkins, Philadelphia

Polit D, Hungler B (1999) *Nursing Research: Principles and methods.* 6th edn. Lippincott Williams & Wilkins, Philadelphia, Pennsylvania

Polit D, Beck C, Hungler B (2001) *Essentials of Nursing Research: Methods, appraisal and utilization.* 5th edn. Lippincott, Philadelphia, Pennsylvania

Porteus S (1892) Posture in parturition. *New York Medical Journal* **56**: 153-154

Poschl U (1987) The vertical birthing positions of the Trobrianders, Papua New Guinea. *Australian and New Zealand Journal of Obstetrics & Gynaecology* **27**(2): 120-125

Price S (1998) Birth plans and their impact on midwifery care. *MIDIRS Midwifery Digest* **8**(2): 189-191

Prince J, Adams M (1987) *The Psychology of Childbirth.* 2nd edn. Churchill Livingstone, New York

Quine L, Rutter D (1996) Birth experiences. In: Niven C, Walker A (Eds) *Conception, Pregnancy and Birth.* Butterworth-Heninemann, Oxford

Racinet C, Eymery P, Philibert L, Lucas C (1999) Labour in the squatting position: a randomized trial comparing the squatting position with the classical position for the expulsion phase. *Journal de Gynecologie, Obstetrique et Biologie de la Reproduction* **28**(3): 263-270

Radkey A, Liston R, Scott K, Young C (1991) Squatting: preventive medicine in childbirth? *Proceedings of the Annual Meeting of the Society of Obstetricians and Gynaecologists of Canada.* Toronto, Ontario: 76

Rapp R (1993) Accounting for amniocentesis. In: Lindenbaum S, Lock M (Eds) *Knowledge, Power and Practice – The anthropology of medicine and everyday life.* University of California Press, Berkeley: 55-79

Redman S, Oak S, Booth P et al (1991) Evaluation of an antenatal education programme: characteristics of attenders, changes in knowledge and satisfaction of participants. *Australian and New Zealand Journal of Obstetrics and Gynaecology* **31**(4): 310-316

Rees C (1996) Antenatal education, health promotion and the midwife. In: Alexander J, Levy V, Roch S (Eds) *Midwifery Practice Core Topic 1.* Macmillan Press, Basingstoke: 58-76

Reynolds J (1991) Primitive delivery positions in modern obstetrics. *Canadian Family Physician* **37**: 356-359

Rhodes L (1990) Studying biomedicine as a cultural system In: Johnson T, Sargent C (Eds) *Medical Anthropology: A handbook of theory and method.* Greenwood Press, Westport

Rigby E (1857) What is the natural position of a woman in labour? *Medical Times & Gazette* **15**: 345-346

Roberts J (1980) Alternative positions for childbirth – second stage of labour. *Journal of Nurse-Midwifery* **25**(5): 13-19

Roberts J, Mendez-Bauer C, Woodell D (1983) The effects of maternal position on uterine contractility. *Birth* **10**(4): 243-249

Robertson A (1994) *Empowering Women: Teaching active birth in the 90s.* Ace Graphics, Australia

Robertson A (1999) When you've got a problem... *Practising Midwife* **2**(7): 46-47

Robertson A (2000) Education for 'Informed choice'. *Practising Midwife* **3**(5): 36-37

Robinson J (2001) Consent for emergency caesareans. *British Journal of Midwifery* **9**(7): 452

Robinson S (1994) Professional development in midwifery: findings from a longitudinal study of midwives' careers. *Nurse Education Today* **4**(3): 161-176

Rogers E (1973) *Communication Strategies For Family Planning.* The Free Press, New York

Rogers E (1983) *Diffusion of Innovations.* 3rd edn. The Free Press, New York

Rogers E (1995) *Diffusion of Innovations.* 4th edn. The Free Press, New York

Rogers E, Kincaid D (1981) *Communication Networks: Toward a New Paradigm for Research.* The Free Press, New York

Rolls C, Cutts D (2001) Pregnancy-to-parenting education: creating a new approach. *Birth* **10**(2): 53-59

Rosser A (1983) Position is everything. *Nursing Times* **79**(44): 42-43

Rothman B (1991) *In Labor: Women and Power in the Birth Place.* Norton, New York

Rotter J (1966) Generalized expectancies for internal versus external control of reinforcement. *Psychological Monographs* **80**(1):1-28

Russell J (1982) The rationale of primitive delivery positions. *British Journal of Obstetrics and Gynaecology* **89**(9): 712-715

Sagady M (2000) The preventable caesarean section: new distinctions and new possibilities. *International Journal of Childbirth Education* **15**(3): 28-31

Sarantakos J (1998) *Social Research.* 2nd edn. Macmillan Press, Basingstoke

Sargent C, Bascope G (1996) Ways of knowing about birth in three cultures. *Medical Anthropology Quarterly* **10**(2): 213-236

Savage W (*1986) A Savage Enquiry – Who controls childbirth, birth & power?* Virago, London

Schott J (1994) The importance of encouraging women to think for themselves. *British Journal of Midwifery* **2**(1): 3-4

Schott J (2003) Antenatal education changes and future developments. *British Journal of Midwifery* **11**(10): S15-S17

Schott J, Henley H (1996) *Culture, Religion and Childbearing in a Multiracial Society.* Butterworth-Heinemann, Oxford

Schott J, Priest J (2002) *Leading Antenatal Classes: A practical guide.* 2nd edn. Butterworth-Heinemann, Oxford

Schwarcz R, Diaz R, Fescina R, Caldeyro-Barcia (1977) Latin American collaborative study on maternal posture in labour. Reported in *Birth and Family Journal* (1979) **6**(1): 22-31

Scott C (2001) Mother's little helpers. In: Dr Foster. *The Good Birth Guide.* The Sunday Times Magazine, 15 July 2001. The Sunday Times Press, UK

Sheer B (1996) Reaching collaboration through empowerment: a developmental process. *Journal of Obstetric, Gynecologic and Neonatal Nursing* **25**(6): 513-517

Shermer R, Raines D (1997) Positioning during the second stage of labor: moving back to basics. *Journal of Obstetric, Gynecologic and Neonatal Nursing* **26**(6), 727-734

Sherr L (1989) Communication and anxiety in obstetric care. Cited in: Sherr L (1995) *The Psychology of Pregnancy and Childbirth.* Blackwell Science, Oxford: 91-114

Shorten A, Donsante J, Shorten B (2002) Birth position, accoucheur and perineal outcomes: informing women about choices for vaginal birth. *Birth* **29**(1):18-27

Shorter E (1991) A typical birth then. In: *A Social History of Women's Encounter with Health, Ill Health and Medicine.* Transaction Publishers, New Jersey, US: 48-68

Simkin P (1991) Just another day in a woman's life? Women's long-term perceptions of their first birth experience. *Birth* **18**(4): 203-210

Simkin P, Enkin M (1989) Antenatal classes. In: Chalmers I, Enkin M, Keirse J (Eds) *A Guide to Effective Care in Pregnancy and Childbirth.* Oxford University Press, Oxford

Slade P (1996) Antenatal preparation. In: Niven C, Walker A (Eds) *Conception, Pregnancy and Birth*. Butterworth-Heinemann, Oxford: 101-113

Slade P, MacPherson S, Hume A, Maresh M (1993) Expectations, experiences and satisfaction with labour. *British Journal of Clinical Psychology* **32**(Pt 4): 469-483

Sleep J (1990) Spontaneous delivery. In: Alexander J, Levy V, Roch S (Eds) *Intrapartum Care: A research-based approach*. Macmillan Education, Basingstoke: 122-136

Sleep J, Roberts J, Chalmers I (1989) Care during the second stage of labour. In: Chalmers I, Enkin M, Keirse MJNC (Eds) *Effective Care in Pregnancy and Childbirth, Volume 2*. Oxford University Press, Oxford: 1129–1144

Smart T (1997) Data analysis. In: Smith P, Hunt J (Eds) *Research Mindedness for Practice*. Churchill Livingstone, New York: 77-113

Soanes C (2000) *The Oxford Compact English Dictionary*. 2nd edn. Oxford University Press, UK

Soot L, Moneta G, Edwards J (1999) Vascular surgery and the internet: a poor source of patient-oriented information. *Journal of Vascular Surgery* **30**(1): 84-91

Sophocles (400 BC) Quoted in: Rogers E (1995) The innovative decision process. In: *Diffusion of Innovations*. 4th edn. The Free Press, New York, US: 161-203

Spinelli A, Baglio G, Donati S et al (2003) Do antenatal classes benefit the mother and her baby? *Journal of Maternal-Fetal and Neonatal Medicine* **13**(2): 94-101

Stapleton H (1997) Choice in the face of uncertainty. In: Kirkham M, Perkins E (Eds) *Reflections of Midwifery*. Baillière Tindall, London: 47-69

Stapleton S (1998) Team building: making collaborative practice work. *Journal of Nurse-Midwifery* **43**(1): 12-18

Starr P (1982) *The Social Transformation of American Medicine*. Basic Books, New York

Stewart P, Hillan E, Calder A (1983) A randomised trial to evaluate use of the birth chair for delivery. *Lancet* **1**: 1296-1298

Stewart P, Spiby H (1989a) A randomised study of the sitting position for delivery using a newly designed obstetric chair. *British Journal of Obstetrics and Gynaecology* **96**(3): 327-333

Stewart P, Spiby H (1989b) Posture in labour. *British Journal of Obstetrics and Gynaecology* **96**(11): 1258-1260

Stichler J (1995) Professional interdependence: the art of collaboration. *Advanced Practice Nursing Quarterly* **1**(1): 53-61

Standing Maternity and Midwifery Advisory Committee (1970) *Domiciliary Midwifery and Maternity Bed Needs: Report of a sub-committee* (The Peel Report). HMSO, London

Strauss A (1987) *Qualitative Analysis for Social Scientists*. Cambridge University Press, Cambridge

Stucky JP (1965) *Der Gerbärstuhl: Die Gründe Für Sein Verschwinden Im Deutschen Sprachbereich*. Juris, Zurich

Sturrock W, Johnson J (1990) The relationship between childbirth education classes and obstetric outcome. *Birth* **17**(2): 82-85

Sudman S, Bradburn M (1982) *Asking Questions: A Practical Guide to Questionnaire Design*. Josey-Bass, San Francisco, California

Symonds A, Hunt C (1996) *The Midwife and Society: Perspectives, Policies and Practice*. Macmillan, London

Tew M (1990) *Safer Childbirth? A critical history of maternity care*. Chapman and Hall, London

The Holy Bible (NIV) (2004) Exodus 1:16, Exodus, New International Version (NIV), International Bible Society, Zondervan Publishers. http://www.bible.gospelcom.net (accessed 13 October 2004)

Thomas R (1996) Surveys. In: Greenfield T (Ed) *Research Methods: Guidance for postgraduates*. Arnold, London: 115-124

Thompson C (1957) *Sidelights on the History of Medicine*. Butterworth & Co, Oxford

Thomson A (1988) Management of the woman in the normal second stage of labour. *Midwifery* **4**(2): 77-85

Thomson A (1993) Pushing techniques in the second stage of labour. *Journal of Advanced Nursing* **8**(2): 171-177

Thomson A (1995) Maternal behaviour during spontaneous and directed pushing in the second stage of labour. *Journal of Advanced Nursing* **22**(6): 1027-1034

Timm M (1979) Prenatal education evaluation. *Nursing Research* **28**(6): 338–342

Tindall VR (1995) *Women in Normal Labour*. Report of a Clinical Standards Advisory Group Committee. HMSO, London

Towler J, Bramall J (1986) *Midwives in History and Society*. Croom Helm, London

Treece E, Treece J (1986) *Elements of Research in Nursing*. 4th edn. CV Mosby, St Louis, US

Turner M, Mona L, Romney J et al (1986) The birthing chair: an obstetric hazard. *Journal of Obstetrics and Gynaecology* **6**: 232-235

UCLA (2001) Training and Consulting Statistical Computing. SPSS FAQ at http://www.oac. ucla.edu/stat/spss/faq/alpha.html (acessed 1 November 2001)

Wagstaff P (2000) Surveys. In: Cluett E, Bluff R (Eds) *Principles and Practice of Research in Midwifery*. Baillière Tindall, Harcourt Publishing, Edinburgh: 11-26

Waldenstrom U, Gottval K (1991) A randomised trial of birthing stool or conventional semi-recumbent position for the 2nd stage of labour. *Birth* **18**(1): 5-10

Wallston K, Wallston B, Smith S, Dobbins C (1987) Perceived control and health. *Current Psychological Research and Reviews* **6**(1): 5-25

Walsh D (1998) Birth positions in a large consultant unit. *The Practising Midwife* **1**(6): 34-36

Walsh D (2000) Why we should reject the 'bed birth' myth. *British Journal of Midwifery* **8**(9): 554-570

Walsh D, Harris M, Shuttlewood S (1999) Changing midwifery birthing practice through audit. *British Journal of Midwifery* **7**(7): 432-435

Walters D, Kirkham M (1997) Support and control in labour: doulas and midwives. In: Kirkham M, Perkins E (Eds) *Reflections on Midwifery*. Baillière Tindall, London: 96-113

Wanless Report (2004) *Securing Good Health for the Whole Population*. Expectations for the Health Service, Chapter 2, http://www.hmtreasury.gov.uk/consultations_and_legislation/ wanless/consult_ wanless04_final.cfm (accessed 4 October 2004)

Weaver J (1998) Choice, control and decision-making. In: Clement S (Ed) *Psychological Perspectives on Pregnancy and Childbirth*. Churchill Livingstone, Edinburgh: 81-99

Weindler G (1915) Geburts und Wochenbetts-Darstellungen auf alt-Agyptischen Tempelreliefs Fig 13. Munich, Bechsche. Cited in: Housholder M (1974) A historical perspective on the obstetric chair. *Surgery, Gynecology and Obstetrics* **139**: 424

Whitford H, Hillan E (1998) Women's perceptions of birthplans. *Midwifery* **14**(4): 248-253

Williams M, Booth D (1985) *Antenatal Education Guidelines for Teachers*. Churchill Livingstone, Edinburgh

World Health Organization (1999) *Care in Normal Birth: A practical guide*. Report of a Technical Working Group. Department of Reproductive Health and Research, WHO, Geneva. http://www.who.int (accessed 11 July 2001)

Wolf von B (1988) The role of cultural, medico-historical traditions on labour and birth position. *Zentrablatt Klinikal Medizine* **43**(19): 1689-1693

Wood S (2003) Should women be given a choice about fetal assessment in labor? *MCN. The American Journal of Maternal Child Nursing* **28**(5): 292-298

Yeoh J, Morrissey C (1996) Selection of library services by post-registration nursing, midwifery and health visiting students. *Health Libraries Review* **13**(2): 97-107

Young A (1982) The anthropologies of illness and sickness. *Annual Review of Anthropology* **11**: 257-285

Index